OVEREATERS ANONYMOUS

THIRD EDITION

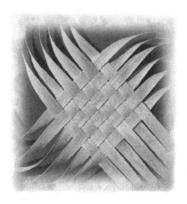

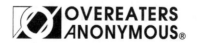

ON THE COVER

"By now OA had completely woven itself into the fabric of my life."
— Rozanne S., *Overeaters Anonymous, Third Edition*, p. 15.

The original photograph and cover design is inspired by Overeaters Anonymous members who gather worldwide to share experiences and find strength and recovery. The twelve strips of woven burlap signify the Twelve Steps and Twelve Traditions and the unity of OA Fellowship. This represents an expression of welcome and hope to all.

Together we can.

Overeaters Anonymous, Inc.

World Service Office

PO Box 44727, Rio Rancho NM 87174-4727 USA

1-505-891-2664

www.oa.org

Second Edition 2001.

Third Edition 2014.

Second Printing 2021.

Printed in the United States of America.

Library of Congress Catalog Card No.: 2014945657

ISBN: 978-1-889681-04-7

CONTENTS

CONTENTS

PREFACE

This is the third edition of *Overeaters Anonymous*, OA's beloved Brown Book. This edition presents forty new recovery stories written by individual OA members. In addition, a new foreword and appendix have been written by non-OA health care professionals who have supported our Fellowship over the last three decades. Other portions of the book remain much the same as in the first and second editions, including the original foreword, "Our Invitation to You," Rozanne's Story, and the original appendices.

FOREWORD

TO THE THIRD EDITION

In 2010, Overeaters Anonymous celebrated its 50th Anniversary at its World Service Convention. As someone who has treated compulsive overeaters for more than three decades, I was privileged to be invited to join in the celebration.

My professional experience with OA dates back to my earlier years in practice, when I began to refer many of my patients to the local OA groups in my area. Doing so left me indebted to the courageous members of this Fellowship who taught me more about this disease than I could have imagined. Since that time, Overeaters Anonymous has been an indispensable support for those who have come to our facility seeking treatment.

I have long believed Overeaters Anonymous serves as a program of ongoing recovery not only for those who suffer from compulsive overeating but also for those who struggle with similar eating disorders. I've continued to witness the success of countless people working the same Twelve Steps, adapted from Alcoholics Anonymous, in OA. Many of my patients, past and present, suffering with bulimia, binge-eating disorder, and related eating disorders have found refuge and recovery at the meetings and among the fellowship OA offers. I believe OA holds a place for anyone wishing to refrain from a compulsive or addictive relationship with food.

I finished my training as a clinical psychologist in 1979, passed my boards, and began a practice specializing in the treatment of eating disorders. Over the next several years, I treated people with various types of eating disorders, most notably compulsive overeating, bulimia, and what is now termed binge-eating disorder. I discovered over time that weight was simply the symptom, and the disease was really an addictive relationship with food and/or dieting.

I say this because I saw people at the university's clinic who were not overweight, yet clearly ate compulsively. Most of these people compensated for their overeating by making themselves sick to get rid of the food, overexercising, or alternating between periods of copious overeating followed by restricting, also known as dieting.

Of course, the majority of folks coming to our program suffered with varying degrees of obesity, the *symptom* most people identify with compulsive overeating. Despite this, I soon concluded that the more appropriate measure of the problem lies with the physical, emotional, and spiritual consequences and not the number on a bathroom scale. In effect, compulsive overeaters had more in common with their alcoholic and drug-addicted brethren than most realized. There was more to this than a "weight problem." In fact, today we see many members of other Twelve Step programs who are also compulsive overeaters and attend OA meetings as part of their ongoing recovery programs.

Not so different from the misguided beliefs about alcoholism in years past, the professional community is currently divided as to how to view, let alone treat, compulsive overeating and related eating disorders. It comes down to those who view compulsive eaters as suffering from a psychiatric illness coupled with a lack of discipline and those who see it as an addictive disease.

Historically, a small group of researchers, physicians, and healthcare professionals have held steadfast to the addiction thesis. I'm pleased to report this minority group of professionals is multiplying and gaining momentum. Recent advances in brain mapping technology such as MRI imaging have clearly identified specific chemical responses in the brain that differentiate a compulsive overeater from his or her "non-addict" peers. The evidence has taken speculation and theory to the level of scientific fact. Personally, this has served to validate myself and those of us who have supported OA through the years—believing that compulsive overeating deserves to be recognized the same way we've come to understand and treat alcoholism and drug addiction.

My experience has shown that active participation in a Twelve Step program such as OA is indispensable to the ongoing success of anyone wishing to recover from compulsive overeating or a similar eating disorder. Although not intended as a substitute for professional treatment, OA affords the best opportunity to gain and keep a foothold in recovery. To help make this point, I'd like to quote from the American Society of Addiction Medicine as it defines the disease of addiction. One can substitute the phrase "compulsive overeating" to see clearly that the proverbial shoe fits.

∿   "Addiction is a primary, chronic disease of brain reward, motivation, memory and related circuitry. Dysfunction in these circuits leads to characteristic biological, psychological, social and spiritual manifestations. This is reflected in an individual pathologically pursuing reward and/or relief by substance use and other behaviors.

Addiction is characterized by inability to consistently abstain, impairment in behavioral control, craving, diminished recognition of significant problems with one's behaviors and interpersonal relationships, and a dysfunctional emotional response. Like other chronic diseases, addiction involves cycles of relapse and remission. Without treatment or engagement in recovery activities, addiction is progressive and can result in disability or premature death."

— American Society Of Addiction Medicine, website, 2013 (www.asam.org)

Just about anyone who attends a support group such as OA for a reasonable period of time will likely hear his or her story told by another member. The effect of one person sharing experiences with a fellow having the same experiences is powerful.

Once the initial layer of the onion is peeled away ("but I'm different than these people"), the stage is set for identification rather than comparison. The question then becomes, "What do I have in common with everyone here? Maybe I'm not alone or so different." From that point forward, the focus begins to center more on the solution: "What do I need to do to recover?"

The "magic" of OA then becomes clear: a combination of people having a common purpose and seeing others working a set of suggested Steps, lending testimony to the promise of recovery.

I hope the Fellowship of OA will continue to grow and its members will continue to serve as a beacon of light for those who have yet to find recovery. It's a spiritual axiom that a group of people with a common history and purpose can do as a group what could not otherwise be achieved by an individual. In that sense, OA offers what no professional or individual person can match: hope by example.

— *Marty Lerner, Ph.D.,* 2013

Dr. Lerner, a clinical psychologist, operates an eating disorder treatment center in Florida. He received the 2010 OA Appreciation Award in recognition of his longtime support of Overeaters Anonymous.

FOREWORD

To the First and Second Editions

I have had both a personal and professional interest in obesity for a great many years. The fact is I've been an overeater all of my life and a fat man most of my life. I did not understand the destructive aspects of overeating, however, until I began to practice psychiatry.

Eventually it became apparent to me that overeating is an obsessive, compulsive addiction of a highly complex nature. I became aware that food can be even more addictive than tobacco, drugs, alcohol, or gambling, and at least as destructive. The simple fact is that we cannot do without food, and each time the food addict eats, he or she is in danger of succumbing to the compulsion.

The further facts are: (1) Food is usually available in abundance. (2) There is no societal, legal dictum against eating. (3) In many places overeating is encouraged. (4) Confusion about this highly complex syndrome abounds.

Indeed, there is still a great deal we do not know about overeating. But we do know now that one's emotional life has a great deal to do with overeating. I believe that repressed anger plays a powerful role in this addiction. I feel that eating binges are often displaced temper tantrums or rage reactions. I also believe that the roots of the condition can often be traced to the earliest times in our lives and to early and complicated family relations. Those who suffer from the problem and those who seriously engage in working in the area also know how malignant the condition is. This destructive aspect occurs relative to the victim's physical health, emotional well-being, social life, professional life, sex life, and economic life.

We also know, unfortunately, how limited all treatment modalities have been to date in effecting sustained relief, let alone "cures." We know, too, how obese people have been patronized, prejudiced against, and exploited for economic gain. Charlatans and chicanery abound. Millions of dollars are made off the suffering of fat people, and this condition is probably the most prevalent health problem that exists in the American population. Of course, as with all other problems, there are varying degrees of difficulty and suffering. But the numbers of people who are driven to seek help make commercial enterprise in this field big business.

Overeaters Anonymous is not a business. This organization represents one of our country's major and perhaps largest efforts at self-help—real and effective self-help. OA enjoys a reputation for significant success in a field strewn with failure. OA's success goes beyond weight reduction and control, though this alone is an achievement of great magnitude. OA also helps to contribute a greater sense of self and self-esteem through its extraordinary implementation of camaraderie and caring for one's fellows and one's self. It functions as a giant contributor to awakening and adding to its members' sense of their own humanity. This is crucial in battling malignant addiction or, for that matter, any illness of the mind and body; they really are one.

This book describes the OA experience as told by various members through their own stories. These are moving and educational stories. They are full of struggle—constructive struggle—and hope. Most important, they tell of enhanced compassion for self, for others, and for the state of being human. They tell us about fellowship and what a powerful therapeutic instrument caring can be. They also tell us what caring is all about. Read them and enjoy being part of the human condition.

— *Theodore Isaac Rubin, M.D.*, 1980

Dr. Rubin is a well-known psychoanalyst practicing psychiatry in New York City. He is past-president of the American Institute for Psychoanalysis and has served on many local and national medical boards. He is the author of more than thirty books, translated worldwide, including *Compassion and Self-Hate, Lisa and David, Jordi, The Winner's Notebook*, and *Lisa and David Today*. Among the many honors he has won are the Adolph Meyer Award from the Association for the Improvement of Mental Health and the Social Conscience Award from the Karen Horney Clinic, a psychiatric institution.

ACKNOWLEDGEMENT

This book would not be possible without our great preceptor, Alcoholics Anonymous. Indeed, many of those whose contributions appear in these pages would not be among us today without the Steps and Traditions of the AA program.

In publishing this collection of personal stories of recovery, Overeaters Anonymous has only one purpose: to describe for all who may be interested the progression of our illness, what we found in this program, and how it has changed us. Our book is not intended as a substitute for or a replacement of *Alcoholics Anonymous*, the life-giving Big Book, which has brought physical, emotional, and spiritual rebirth to millions around the globe.

Those of us who speak in these pages confirm the prophetic words used in 1951 in conferring the Lasker Award on the then sixteen-year-old Fellowship of Alcoholics Anonymous:

"Historians may one day recognize Alcoholics Anonymous to have been a great venture in social pioneering which forged a new instrument for social action; a new therapy based on the kinship of common suffering; one having a vast potential for the myriad other ills of mankind." (*Alcoholics Anonymous*, 4th ed., p. 573)

Our deepest gratitude to the Fellowship of Alcoholics Anonymous for their continued growth without promotion, exemplary leadership without leaders, and principles without personalities.

Our Invitation to You

We of Overeaters Anonymous have made a discovery. At the very first meeting we attended, we learned that we were in the clutches of a dangerous illness, and that willpower, emotional health, and self-confidence, which some of us had once possessed, were no defense against it.

To be sure, the picture painted of the disease was grim: progressive, debilitating, incurable. Compulsive eating has many symptoms in addition to mere fat. It is also an illness that isolates and gradually, or rapidly, causes increasingly serious problems in one or more areas of our lives: health, job, finances, family, or social life.

No one is sure what causes it, probably a number of factors: environment, a certain way of reacting to life, biological predisposition.

We have learned that the reasons are unimportant. What deserves the attention of the still-suffering compulsive overeater is this: There is a proven, workable method by which we can arrest our illness.

The OA recovery program is patterned after that of Alcoholics Anonymous. As the personal stories in this book attest, the Twelve

Step program of recovery works as well for compulsive eaters as it does for alcoholics. Our members prove that compulsive eaters can share their problems and help each other, thus benefiting not only themselves but their families and the communities in which they live.

Can we guarantee you this recovery? The answer is up to you. If you will honestly face the truth about yourself and the illness; if you will keep coming back to meetings to talk and listen to other recovering compulsive overeaters; if you will read our literature and that of Alcoholics Anonymous with an open mind; and, most important, if you are willing to rely on a Power greater than yourself for direction in your life and to take the Twelve Steps to the best of your ability, we believe you can indeed join the ranks of those who recover.

The disease of compulsive eating causes or contributes to illness on three levels—emotional, physical, and spiritual. To remedy this threefold illness we offer several suggestions, but the reader should keep in mind that the basis of the program is spiritual, as evidenced by the Twelve Steps.

We are not a "diet club." We do not endorse any particular plan of eating. In OA, abstinence is the act of refraining from compulsive eating and compulsive food behaviors while working towards or maintaining a healthy body weight. Once we become abstinent, the preoccupation with food diminishes and in many cases leaves us entirely. We then find that, to deal with our inner turmoil, we have to have a new way of thinking, of acting on life rather than reacting to it—in essence, a new way of living.

From this vantage point, we begin OA's Twelve Step program of recovery, moving beyond the food and the emotional havoc to a fuller living experience.

We believe that no amount of willpower or self-determination could have saved us. Times without number, our resolutions and plans were shattered as we saw our individual resources fail.

So we honestly admitted to ourselves that we were powerless over food. This was the first step toward recovery. It followed that, if we had no power of our own, we needed a power outside ourselves to help us recover.

Some of us, including agnostics and atheists, regard the group itself as a power greater than ourselves. Others choose to accept different interpretations of this power. But most of us adopt the concept of God as God may be understood by each individual.

As a result of practicing the Steps, the symptoms of compulsive eating and compulsive food behaviors are removed on a daily basis. Thus, for most of us, abstinence means freedom from the bondage of compulsive overeating, achieved through the process of surrendering to something greater than ourselves; the more total our surrender, the more fully realized our freedom from food obsession.

Here are the Steps as adapted for Overeaters Anonymous:

1. We admitted we were powerless over food—that our lives had become unmanageable.

2. Came to believe that a Power greater than ourselves could restore us to sanity.

3. Made a decision to turn our will and our lives over to the care of God *as we understood Him.*

4. Made a searching and fearless moral inventory of ourselves.

5. Admitted to God, to ourselves and to another human being the exact nature of our wrongs.

6. Were entirely ready to have God remove all these defects of character.

7. Humbly asked Him to remove our shortcomings.

8. Made a list of all persons we had harmed, and became willing to make amends to them all.

9. Made direct amends to such people wherever possible, except when to do so would injure them or others.

10. Continued to take personal inventory and when we were wrong, promptly admitted it.

11. Sought through prayer and meditation to improve our conscious contact with God *as we understood Him*, praying only for knowledge of His will for us and the power to carry that out.

12. Having had a spiritual awakening as the result of these Steps, we tried to carry this message to compulsive overeaters and to practice these principles in all our affairs.*

*Permission to use the Twelve Steps of Alcoholics Anonymous for adaptation granted by AA World Services, Inc.

"How can I face this?" you may ask. We suggest you do so only one day at a time. "Just for today" is one of many deeply meaningful OA slogans. "I can do anything for twenty-four hours that I couldn't do for a lifetime" was a brand new way of thinking for us. Before, we looked at our weight problem—and all our other problems—and said, "What's the use? It's too much for me. I can't possibly do it."

Now, we fully accept and live by the premise that we don't have to look at everything all at once. We know that it's necessary to do a certain amount of planning, but once having planned, we act for this one day alone.

"But I'm too weak. I'll never make it!" Don't worry; we have all thought and said the same thing. The amazing secret to the success of this program is just that: weakness. It is weakness, not strength, that binds us to each other and to a Higher Power and somehow gives us an ability to do what we cannot do alone. We have discovered that if people in this program love us, it is not for our strength, but for our weakness and our willingness to share that with others.

After reading the personal stories in this book, you may proclaim, "I'm not that bad!" Once again, we ask you to keep in mind that compulsive eating is a progressive illness. If you really are a compulsive eater, the symptoms will grow worse. Within our ranks are those who were recovering but tried once again to control food by their own devices, with consequent return to serious compulsive eating and, in many cases, massive weight gain, starving, or purging.

If you can identify with the developing pattern of uncontrollable eating revealed in our stories, you probably are a compulsive overeater. The chances are that your symptoms will eventually reach those of late-stage compulsive eating. In other words, you're not that bad—yet!

If, after reading this book, you decide you are one of us, we welcome you with open arms. You are not alone anymore! Overeaters Anonymous extends to all of you the gift of acceptance. No matter who you are, where you come from, or where you are going, you are welcome here. Regardless of what you have done or failed to do, what you have felt or haven't felt, who you have loved or hated, you may be sure of our unconditional acceptance.

We will help you and rejoice with you and tell you that we are not failures just because we sometimes fail. We'll hold out our arms in love and stand beside you as you pull yourself back up and walk on again to where you are heading.

Sometimes we fail to be all that we could be, and sometimes we aren't there to give you all you need from us. Accept our imperfections, too. Love and help us in return. That is what we are in OA— imperfect but progressing. Let us rejoice together in our recovery and in the assurance that we have a home, if we want it.

Welcome to Overeaters Anonymous. Welcome home!

1

KEEP COMING BACK: ROZANNE'S STORY

ROZANNE S., OA'S FOUNDER, SHARES HER STORY
OF THE FELLOWSHIP'S EARLIEST DAYS.

Honey, if you have a 23-inch (59 cm) waist, everything else will be all right." My mother's words were to haunt me all my growing-up years. The promise that a slender figure would bring instant and permanent happiness was an illusion in which I believed with all my heart. The few times I was thin, nothing else changed. I thought that the fault was mine. "If only I tried harder," I told myself, "everything would be different." The persistence of my illusion was astonishing.

Trying harder was our family tradition. I come from a family of superachievers and compulsive overeaters. My mother grew up in Green Bay, Wisconsin, in the early 1900s. In that small town my grandfather owned the first movie theaters and the first automobile. My grandmother was very daring for those times—she supported Margaret Sanger several years before Sanger founded Planned Parenthood. My father was world famous in his own right in B'nai B'rith, an international Jewish organization. My mother was one of

America's first dieticians in the early 1920s.

My parents were loving perfectionists, and both were extremely education oriented. My younger brother and I learned early that the way to be worth anything was to work very hard and to achieve beyond the scope of most other people. Growing up, we believed that just being a loving person wasn't enough; we had to excel to be worthwhile.

In my very early teens, I decided I wanted to be a famous actress, pretending to be someone else, noticed and applauded for my efforts and talent. Maybe then I would be acceptable.

Born in Milwaukee, Wisconsin, I moved with my family to Chicago when I was twelve. Sadly, I'd been an overweight child, and now I was becoming a very pudgy teenager. Often I heard well-meaning people say, "You have such a pretty face, dear. If only you'd lose weight." That broke my heart. Did it mean I wasn't any good because I was fat? I just tried a little harder, worked a little more, studied a little longer.

None of it had any effect. You see, buried in my soul was the secret I told no one—I hated myself—and no amount of superachieving could bring me peace of mind.

As I entered my third year at the University of Chicago, I had just turned 18. It seemed that all the other girls were dating, but I was alone in my dorm room on Saturday nights. It was obvious that being fat would never attract boys, so I made a decision to give up overeating. At 142 pounds (64 kg), I went on a diet, and for the first time in my life I became thin. I was 5 feet 2 inches (157 cm) and weighed 118 pounds (54 kg).

Suddenly the boys began to notice me. I had so many dates, I began to neglect my studies and flunked every subject. I can still feel my parents' anger and disappointment. My furious father insisted on sending me to business school. "Not only will you learn your lesson," he said, "but you'll gain some skills with which to earn a living." (It was this excellent training that prepared me for setting up the first OA office in my dining room ten years later.) Unfortunately, I returned to overeating and regained all the weight I had lost. The following year I returned to put myself through the University and earn a BA degree.

After graduation, I began working as a producer's secretary in a local summer theater. There I met Imogene Coca, a famous television comedienne. I told her I was going to New York City in the fall to find work in the theater or television. "Be sure to call me," she urged, "and I'll help you find a job." My famous friend kept her word, and I soon found myself working as a producer's secretary at NBC on TV specials with Bob Hope, Eddie Cantor, and Kate Smith.

In that position, I could see the constant rejections received by auditioning actors and actresses. My own fear of rejection was so strong that it overrode my lifelong acting ambition. I settled for working behind the scenes as a producer's secretary, where it was safe.

Those were the early days of commercial television, an exciting life for a young woman. Still I had no peace of mind. At 142 pounds (64 kg), I hated my body, but I couldn't seem to stop overeating.

In addition, I had developed a fierce resentment toward my mother and now blamed her for my unhappiness. (Years later, after much Twelve Step work on myself, that resentment was removed, and I finally took responsibility for my own actions.)

After two years I returned home to Chicago, where I became a fashion copywriter at a large department store. At last I had found my lifelong vocational love: writing.

But youth is restless. My mother's mother lived in sunny Los Angeles, and I sensed an opportunity. "I've had enough of winter snow," I told my mother. "I'm going to California to live with Grandma and to find fame, fortune, and a husband." In Los Angeles I again went to great lengths to find a boyfriend—I gave up excess food and became slender once more. After another copywriting stint, I became assistant advertising manager of a prestigious chain of department stores. The job was terrific, I was thin, men were calling me for dates, and life really seemed to be going my way.

Yet something was terribly wrong. What was it? No matter what happened, no matter how tiny I was, self-hate still ate at my very soul. I couldn't even admit it to myself.

In January 1955, I joined my girlfriend at a Sunday afternoon charity dance at the famous Ambassador Hotel. "Oh, look," said my friend, pointing across the room. "There's Marv S____. I dated him once. Come on, I'll introduce you."

After exchanging names, I looked up into the kindest eyes I'd ever seen. Smiling down at me was Marvin, my gentle, caring partner-to-be. I was 26 years old, I weighed 118 pounds (54 kg), I was falling in love. Despite such wonders, I was barely hanging onto my diet. Old feelings still raged underneath, and old habits were biding their time, waiting for the crack in my armor.

Marvin proposed to me in August, and at our wedding four months later, I weighed 129 pounds (59 kg). All it took was that little ring on my finger for me to take back the food.

That was only the beginning. Ten months later Debbie was born, and Julie came along 17 months after that. By this time, life was too much for me. I weighed 148 pounds (67 kg), with more fat piling on every day. I couldn't stop eating, and most of the time I wished I were dead. My self-worth was completely gone, my soul was empty, I had no place to go, and I didn't believe in God. What was left for me?

The answer came late one quiet November night in 1958. Marvin and my babies were asleep, and it was time for my usual routine of TV watching and eating. Twenty-nine years old and 152 pounds (69 kg), I spent every night until bedtime filling my inner emptiness with excess food.

Paul Coates, a syndicated television journalist, hosted a weekly show called Paul Coates' Confidential File. That night he was interviewing a member from a new organization called Gamblers Anonymous. My husband had a friend who was a compulsive gambler, and I thought this might be just the thing for him. So Marvin and I took his friend to a GA meeting just before Thanksgiving.

As long as I live, I will never forget that night. We were in a meeting hall with about twenty-five men and a sprinkling of wives. Each man in turn got up and talked about his life of lying and cheating, stealing and hiding. Sitting in the back of that room with my big, black coat clutched around me, I was absolutely transfixed. "I'm just like that," I said to myself. "Their compulsion is with gambling and mine is with food, but now I know I'm not alone anymore!" I discovered that I wasn't wicked or sinful; I was sick. I had an illness, and I could give it a name—compulsive overeating. It was a revelation, and when I walked out of the meeting room that night, my life changed forever.

I wanted to talk to other overeaters, but I couldn't find any groups for people like me. Terrified, I didn't know where to turn. Years of conventional therapy had not helped my compulsive overeating. Where could I go? What should I do?

Clinging to a diet for the next three weeks, I finally gave in and went back to my old ways. Helpless and hopeless, I didn't know that I needed other people for support and a life-changing program for recovery.

I continued to overeat and cry for another year. In November 1959, new neighbors moved in down the block. The woman, Jo S., weighed over 200 pounds (91 kg), and I'd never seen anyone who looked like her. When I saw her, I said to myself, "I'll never look like that. I'll never let myself weigh that much." Aren't those famous last words for an overeater?

Now, approaching a new year, I was only 30 years old, and I was fatter than I'd ever been. During the holidays, I had gained nine pounds (4 kg) in a week and a half! Now weighing 161 pounds (73 kg), I wore a size 20. I'd never weighed that much, never been that fat. Yet that was the catalyst that propelled me into action.

Despairing and desperate, I remembered that night at Gamblers Anonymous. I told my husband, "Marvin, I can't find any group, so I'm going back to Gamblers Anonymous to see if it's the same as I remember."

By late 1959, GA was two and a half years old; several of the men I'd heard before were still there, and they welcomed me warmly.

After the meeting, I approached Jim W., the founder of Gamblers Anonymous. It must have been quite a sight—a 5-foot-2-inch

(157 cm), overweight, young woman staring up into the face of a 6-foot-2-inch (188 cm), skinny, middle-aged man.

Heart pounding, I asked, "Jim, do you think an organization like yours could work for compulsive overeaters like me?" He smiled down at me gently. "I don't see why not. I was in Alcoholics Anonymous before I started GA."

There it was—a hand outstretched to steady me as I stumbled along. It was my first experience with the Twelfth Step, the first time anyone had offered to help me with no thought of reward. I went home and told Marvin, "I think I finally have a chance."

From the moment the idea occurred to me, I envisioned a Fellowship as big as AA or bigger, with meetings all around the world. "If the alcoholic is a compulsive overdrinker," I mused to myself, "then we must be compulsive overeaters. I'll call our organization Overeaters Anonymous."

Meanwhile, Christmas came and went. One crisp December afternoon I was strolling my babies down the block when I spied my overweight neighbor wheeling her baby across the street. "Here's my chance," I said to myself. "It's now or never!"

I joined her, and we chatted for a few minutes. As we approached my house, I blurted out, "Jo, I've got to rush. I have to go to the health club to see about starting this group."

"This group? What group?" she asked. "Well," I answered, "I know you don't share this problem, but I'm a compulsive overeater, and I'm having a terrible time."

Intrigued, she persisted. "What's the name of your group?"

I took a deep breath. "Overeaters Anonymous."

"You know," she offered, "I would be interested. I think I'd like to try it with you." At that moment, the Fellowship of Overeaters Anonymous was born.

I was elated and filled with hope. "Maybe I'll have a chance now," I said to myself. "I won't be alone anymore."

A few days later, during a physical checkup, my doctor said, "Rozanne, you need to lose about 50 pounds (23 kg). I have just the pill to help you lose weight." Remember, this was the beginning of the 1960s. Along with many others, I was naive regarding drugs, and I viewed my doctor as The Authority. Overstimulated as a result of the medicine, I stopped excessive eating, and for six months I had the cleanest house in Los Angeles! During that period, I went from 161 pounds (73 kg) to 120 pounds (54 kg) and eventually to 110 pounds (50 kg), a weight I maintained for several years. However, despite my dramatic weight loss, my heart and soul were still buried in self-hate, and I didn't know how to rescue myself. The medicine helped for the six months I took it, but my efforts to start OA were to be the most important factor in changing both my body and my inner sense of self-esteem.

In addition to my first two visits to GA, Jo accompanied me to one more meeting. Neither of us knew anything about AA. On January 19, 1960, we held the first OA meeting. Jo and I were there, along with Bernice, the wife of a GA member. For all of us, it was a relief to be able to talk about our struggles with someone who understood.

Suddenly, during the start of the third meeting, Bernice said, "My doctor says dieting makes me nervous." With that she got up and walked out the door. Jo and I looked at each other. I was stunned and frightened. Was it over before it had started? Had I lost my only hope? Jo wanted to leave, but I started to cry and said that I couldn't do it alone, insisting that she had to stay. She agreed.

We struggled along. By August we had both lost a lot of weight. Jo went from 200 pounds (91 kg) to 109 pounds (49 kg) in nine months; I came down from 161 pounds (73 kg) to 118 pounds (54 kg) in the same time. Physically, we were splendid examples to prospective members.

However, in the beginning, the less I ate the more my anxieties and feelings of worthlessness rose to the surface. Because I couldn't admit them, even to myself, I covered everything with a lot of self-willed actions.

The first thing I decided was that those AA Steps were very poorly written. "That Bill W. [AA's cofounder] was only a stockbroker," I snickered to myself, "and I'm a professional writer. I can do a better job on the Steps." I thought I knew everything.

In addition, the training in my Jewish home had been more tra-
ditionally ethnic than spiritual. I believed that I was not so weak
that I had to turn my life and my will over to the care of any God,
whether He existed or not. Therefore, I removed AA's Step Three
and wrote a new one.

Because I felt strongly about the importance of nutrition and
calorie-counting, my new Step Three advocated consultation "with
a physician of our own choosing." Adamant and defiant, I proceed-
ed to remove the word "God" and all mention of spiritual concepts
from the rest of the Steps. Then I took a good look at what I had
done and realized that the Steps didn't look at all like those of AA.

"After all," I sighed, "I do want people to say we are like AA." So
I reluctantly sprinkled God back into a few of the Steps. Neither Jo
nor I knew any better.

OA became an integral part of my life from its beginning. I was
obsessed with my vision, living and breathing it as I continued to
care for my home and family. Most important, I had finally found
someone to talk to, someone who understood my struggles with
food.

After a few weeks I read my rewritten Steps to Jim W. He must
have been horrified, but he'd talked to me enough to realize I was
one of those examples of self-will run riot the AA Big Book talks
about. I was starting my own game and making my own rules as I
went along. Biding his time, he said nothing.

In April Barbara S. joined our little group. Now there were Jo
and Barbara and me. Drifting in and out were several friends of
ours. Nobody in our new little group had been to AA. I had been
to three GA meetings; Jo had been to one GA meeting with me.
During our weekly OA meetings we discussed our feelings on a psychological level. We knew nothing of the meaning of inventories
or amends, and I bristled at the thought of surrender and spiritual
awakening.

After a few weeks Jim suggested that we visit an AA meeting.
"Oh, I couldn't," I shot back. "They might be drunk and accost us."

Oh, the patience of Jim!

"No, no," he laughed. "The drunks are in many other places, but the sober ones are in the AA meetings." Trembling inside and very fearful, Jo and I went to an AA meeting.

That was an eye-opening experience for me. I listened to concepts I'd never heard before, and I felt a tangible love in the room. Unfortunately, my fears were in the way, and I was still unable to accept many of the basic precepts of the AA program, especially those contained in the original Twelve Steps. Most important, I refused to embrace the idea of surrendering my life and will to the care of a Higher Power.

The thinner I became and the more I achieved, the worse I felt. I didn't dare let people know this. They might find out how terrible I was. (I remember receiving a standing ovation when I was introduced at our first Conference in 1962. Later I confessed to my sponsor, Thelma, "If they knew how rotten I am, they wouldn't stand up and applaud, they would stand up and turn around and walk out!")

Jo left California and OA in August 1960. That left Barbara and me and five other women who resisted the OA program at every meeting. I was frightened. What would happen to my magnificent dream? By that time I weighed 117 pounds (53 kg), and Barbara had gone down from 192 pounds (87 kg) to 132 pounds (60 kg). Physically, we were both programs of attraction. Finally, Paul Coates interviewed us on his syndicated TV show in November 1960. The show ran in six cities, and we received five hundred letters. By now OA had completely woven itself into the fabric of my life. I couldn't tell where marriage and motherhood ended and OA began. Excited by the telecast, I felt enormous hope for my recovery. Yet, I couldn't admit the uncertainty and fear that often overwhelmed me.

Right after the interview, Jim began urging me to reinstate AA's original Step Three. Stubbornly, I refused. "Listen Rozanne," he coaxed. "If you could have done it by yourself, you would have done it by yourself. But all your life you've depended on doctors, fad diets, and pills. These are all powers outside of you. Now," he went on, "you have a meeting every week, and you talk to someone every day. Don't you see that these are powers outside of you, too?" Reluctantly, I agreed.

His next few statements were to alter my life forever. "Rozanne," he persisted, "suppose you take the capital "p" off of Power and make it a small "p." Then say, 'I'm willpowerless over food.' Can you do that?" With that phrase, Jim had grabbed my attention. "Will-power" was a dieter's term. All my life I'd said, "I have no willpower." Now I could admit to being willpowerless over food without having to admit to a belief in a Higher Power. Without my realizing it, Jim had opened the door to a spiritual way of life for me. I couldn't step over that threshold yet, but the time was coming.

As a result of Jim's insistence, I gave in and wrote some new Twelve Steps. AA's Third Step was reinstated, but I still couldn't make all of our Steps identical to AA's Steps.

During the next two years my own inner conflicts increased. I was not overeating, I was thin, and I was a mass of self-will imposed on everyone. I felt that because I was slender and had been one of OA's founders that every word I uttered was a pearl of wisdom. Everyone ought to listen to me. That was the only way I could make myself feel important. I couldn't achieve that feeling from inside, and I simply didn't know what else to do.

Frequently I stepped on the toes of my fellow members, and they retaliated. Members began vilifying me in the meetings; some even telephoned to call me names. Late one Tuesday night a woman called to read me the riot act in no uncertain terms. Two nights later she did the same thing. She slammed her receiver down; I was helpless and horrified. I threw myself down on the floor in the darkened living room. Sobbing uncontrollably, I cried out, "God, if you're there, you've got me." And that's how I found the God of my understanding.

However, my recovery was only beginning. The resentment toward my mother, which I had carried for twenty-five years, was corroding my very core. "It's time for Steps Eight and Nine," said my sponsor, Thelma. At her prodding, I made amends to my parents. They lived in another city, so I had to write to them. I took the letter to the big mailbox on the corner and dropped it in. As I turned to walk away, I heard the heavy clank of the mailbox door. With that sound, twenty-five years of resentment disappeared. In one brief moment, everything was gone! I could hardly believe it; to me it was a miracle.

My next major step occurred in early 1962. In those days, and while I was growing up, calorie counting had been the dieter's mainstay. That's how I had learned to cut my food intake. It didn't matter how much I ate or how often, as long as my total food count remained within the limits I had set for myself. Unfortunately, nibbling on low-calorie vegetables between meals only increased my compulsion.

Although I'm not an alcoholic, during those early years I was attending AA meetings every week in order to learn more about the Twelve Steps and Twelve Traditions. Late in 1961, one powerful, Sunday, noon AA meeting completely transformed my way of thinking about eating. Ordinarily, the AA members talked about sobriety. However, on this day the main speaker kept referring to "abstinence" from alcohol. This was the first time I'd ever heard sobriety referred to in that manner. It was a revelation!

Sitting in the back row, I said to myself, "That's what wrong with all of us in OA, including me. We're not abstaining from food during the day at all. Nibbling between meals is only reinforcing our obsession. Sometime during the day we have to 'abstain' from eating." Because I am a dietician's daughter, I recalled my mother's teachings about three meals a day.

At the next OA meeting, I was really excited. "Listen, everybody," I bubbled, "I have a new idea. With our between-meal nibbling, we're not abstaining from eating at all. That applies to me as well. We need to close our mouths from the end of one meal to the beginning of the next. I know we have to eat, so let's try three meals a day. We'll have nothing in between but no-calorie beverages, and we'll call that abstinence. If your doctor says more meals, the same principle will apply." Even then I knew abstaining referred not to the food plan itself but to the act of staying away from compulsive eating.

Some members thought it was an inspiration; others just laughed. But many members violently disagreed, and that's when the arguments began. I jumped right into the fight, and the negative excitement threatened to destroy my emerging serenity. However, I was still thin and going to meetings, so I believed I was safe from my disease.

In July 1964, after several inventories, I took one specifically on compulsive spending. On July 30, when I brought the inventory to my sponsor's house, I weighed 109 pounds (49 kg). I walked out of Thelma's home believing that I would never spend like that again. I walked right into a family party, took that first bite, and continued to overeat.

A year later, although my overspending had stopped, my eating was out of control, and I'd gained 17 pounds (8 kg) with no end in sight. Terrified at what was happening to me, I resigned as national secretary. Luckily, Margaret P., a former executive secretary, stepped in to take my place.

Six years later Margaret died of cancer, and I came back to fill her job. Unfortunately, I was fat and getting fatter. By late April 1972, I was back to 148 pounds (67 kg). The trustees fired me as OA's national secretary. They felt that everyone representing OA at the national level had to be a physical example of recovery. To save face, I submitted a letter of resignation, citing ill health and family pressures.

Years later I came to appreciate the value of the trustees' actions. They had not enabled my disease. They had insisted on recovery on all three levels for OA national service workers, and they were absolutely right. I will be forever grateful to them for this valuable lesson.

At that time, however, self-pity overwhelmed me. I took that firing as a personal rejection. Somehow, the essence of the OA program was eluding me, and only food could ease my misery. By the following year, my body ballooned to 185 pounds (84 kg). Confusion and despair filled my life.

Yet, one blessing remained—I kept coming back to meetings.

Sitting in the back of the room, I felt hopeless and desolate, unable to make a phone call when I wanted to eat. Compulsive overeating is a disease of isolation, and my paralyzing inability to call was part of my illness.

Finally, one hot summer night in 1973, I heard a speaker, Cynthia L., whom I'd never seen before. Approaching her after the meeting, I told her I was leaving OA, that this was my last meeting.

The next morning she called me. "Hi, Rozanne, I just wanted to tell you I love you." Cynthia called me every day for weeks. She loved me because I was a member of the human race, not because I was thin or had achieved anything marvelous. Her simple acceptance of me kept me in Overeaters Anonymous.

The next years were a great learning experience for me. Although I began to lose weight very slowly, incomprehensible demoralization was still a part of my daily life. I kept coming back to OA, and I certainly learned a lot about patience. Yet the ability to love myself still eluded me; my heart was clouded with self-hate.

One day in late 1978 during an OA convention meeting, I heard a speaker, Mary, tell her story. As she ended, she said, "I tried to tell myself, 'Mary, you're okay,' and I couldn't say it in front of a mirror. It took me six months to do it."

Later that night I bragged to myself, "I can certainly do that right now." But I couldn't. I tried to tell myself I was okay, and I started to cry. Then I remembered my sponsor's lessons. Thelma had taught me to "act as if." She told me that I didn't have to want it, like it, or believe it. "Just take the action," she had urged, "and the feelings will follow."

Acting as if it were true, I practiced telling myself, "Rozanne, you're okay." Unable to look at myself in the mirror, I said this phrase all day, every day, for six months. Then one December evening, I was dressed for a party. In a hurry to leave, I paused briefly to check myself in the hall mirror before rushing out the door. Then I suddenly stopped and looked at myself. I smiled and said, "Rozanne, you're okay. You are one fantastic lady, and I love you." That wondrous feeling has remained with me to this day, evidence of God's work in my life.

By late 1979 I weighed 137 pounds (62 kg). My family doctor had given me an antidepressant to ease my ever-present headaches, but that particular drug had an unfortunate side effect. It caused weight gain. By September 1981, I was back to 172 pounds (78 kg). Luckily, an eating-disorder specialist discovered my plight and took me off the drug. With that action, some of my overeating lessened and 25 of my excess pounds (11 kg) disappeared.

But still I struggled. Abstaining for short periods, I would give in and overeat again. What was wrong? I prayed for a miracle, terrified that I might be an OA failure, ashamed to return to meetings. Yet I knew there was nowhere else for me to go, and so I kept coming back. Little by little, I gained weight again.

By spring of 1986 I weighed 171 pounds (77 kg). Then slowly I began to abstain from the worst of my compulsive overeating. There were still slips, but surrender gradually entered my heart. I began to truly realize that I was a compulsive overeater who couldn't control her eating alone. I wasn't bingeing as I had in the past; I wasn't eating between my planned meals. Again I prayed for help. Suddenly, the unexpected happened.

In January 1987, the Los Angeles Intergroup had its annual OA birthday party. A.G., my longtime friend from Texas, had returned to OA after an eighteen-year absence. In 1962, he had been the first man in OA. He had lost over 100 pounds (45 kg) and had been chairman of our first Board of Trustees. Then, like so many, he had left OA and regained the weight.

By January 1987, this wonderful man had been back in OA for a year. He was maintaining his normal weight and working the Steps. He came to Los Angeles from his Texas home to join in the birthday celebration.

He and my husband, Marvin, and I went out to dinner each night, taking turns paying the bill. One fateful night A.G. took a piece of paper out of his pocket and began writing.

"What are you doing?" I protested. "It's our turn to pay the bill."

He shook his head and continued writing. "I'm counting my

calories," he replied.

His comment stayed with me all through that night. My treasured friend had what I wanted. He had a slender body, and more important, his eyes had a light that could only come from spiritual recovery.

"If he can make it, I can make it," I told myself. "I grew up counting calories. That's not so scary; I can do that."

Praying for guidance, I asked God for an eating plan I could live with the rest of my life. "Through health and illness, through travel and at home, through parties, bar mitzvahs, holidays, and ordinary days, help me to nourish my body with the right food in the proper amounts." Then I said, "However long it takes to lose this weight is however long it's going to take."

The next day I sat down to write an eating plan for myself. Allowing for several health problems and my age, height, and daily activities, I arrived at a nourishing plan for myself, with abstinence from food between my allotted meals.

That day I began to weigh and measure everything I ate. I hadn't been bingeing in my old manner, but I was appalled at how much I'd been consuming. No wonder I was still fat! At my short height, I was eating too much for my body.

By the third day of this new plan I began to feel a lightening of my spirit, as if an inner weight were being lifted. It was so beautiful; I knew at once it was hope. For the first time in years, I could see the light at the end of the tunnel. Because I'd been going to meetings for twenty-seven years, I understood that I would have to work those Twelve Steps immediately. No matter how effective my eating plan was, weighing and measuring alone just wouldn't work. My salvation lay in those Steps.

I had long ago learned that eating plans and meetings are not my program of recovery. Although they are helpful and even necessary, AA's Big Book statement was more than ever true for me: "Here are the Steps which are suggested as a program of recovery."

Since 1961, I've taken twenty-four Fourth Steps and hundreds of Tenth Steps. Today I continue to surrender, make amends, carry the OA message, and practice these principles in all my affairs.

Beginning in 1962, I've had a period of prayer and meditation every morning before I start my day. It's become a habit, one which has stood me in good stead as I surrendered myself to my Higher Power each day and admitted my powerlessness over food.

Since our recovery is spiritual, emotional, and physical, I'm careful to include a daily routine of exercise and walking. It took three years to lose 40 pounds (18 kg). That slow weight loss allowed my mind to become thin along with my body. (On other diets, I'd lost weight so fast that my head stayed fat while my figure slenderized.)

Because I pay attention to what goes into my mouth, I can pay attention to what goes into my heart and mind and soul. Today I can enjoy a normal-size body while maintaining a 60-pound (27-kg) weight loss from my top weight.

Instead of being a struggle, life is really fun! I delight in spending time with my husband and with my daughters and their husbands. I can take pleasure in playing with my small grandsons and appreciate working in my beautiful rose garden.

I care about others because I care about myself. Because I kept coming back, I learned the validity of an elementary spiritual principle given to me by the Reverend Rollo M. Boas, one of OA's earliest supporters: "If you remove your body from the truth, when you are ready, the truth is nowhere to be found. But if you continue to bring your body to the truth, then when you are ready, the truth is waiting there for you."

And that truth—our promise of recovery—is in every OA meeting when we join hands, pray together, and joyously, lovingly encourage one another: Keep coming back!

A LOVING TRIBUTE

Since this story was written, a heart attack took my beloved husband, Marvin, on November 11, 1999. Many of you knew him well. Most of you have heard me praise his patience, support, and encouragement during OA's first forty years. He took care of our babies when Jo S. and I met during that first year. He strengthened and sustained me when I set up an office in our little dining room. He joined us—you and me—at birthday parties, conferences, and conventions, always sharing in our trials and triumphs. He believed in us and what we were trying to achieve. Marvin was our earliest and most faithful friend, and we will all miss his loving, gentle presence.

IN MEMORIAM

OA's beloved founder, Rozanne S., passed away January 16, 2014. Rozanne's compassion for and understanding of the emotional, physical, and spiritual challenges faced by compulsive eaters have touched people worldwide. She leaves an enduring legacy that will continue to inspire and heal those who still suffer.

For more on the history of Overeaters Anonymous, read *Beyond Our Wildest Dreams*, available in the OA bookstore at www.oa.org.

2

OA THEN AND NOW

I wrote my story for *Overeaters Anonymous, Second Edition* when I was in my early 30s. At the time I had already been in OA half my life. With the help of OA I had grown up and started to enjoy the benefits of living in the program. I was very active in all types of service. I found my talents in life, and that led me to an enjoyable career in business. I had (and still have) a great support system of OA friends who helped me celebrate the successes and get through the losses in my life. I saw that I was truly blessed, even when life didn't seem fair.

During this period, my family relationships healed greatly, and I started to learn to love myself. The people in OA showed me love and acceptance. As I worked the Steps and developed a relationship with a Higher Power, I stopped feeling ashamed of who I was and how awkward I felt. Soon I was able to be alone and enjoy my own company.

It was a miracle for me to choose a career that involved dealing with lots of people, stress, and pressure. I was the same person who grew up with fear and always thought I would be a failure. I learned to take the OA Principles into my workplace. I learned to treat customers and employees the same way I treated fellow OA members. When fear or anger came up, I could use the OA Tools and Steps to deal with them. I had a lot of success at work, but more importantly, I helped other people, mentored employees, and strove to be a living example of the OA program.

I was also blessed to make living amends to my parents and family. I was able to be there for them as they started to age and have health issues. I was fortunate that I didn't yet have my own family, and I could balance working at my career, giving lots of service in OA, and spending time with my parents.

As an example of our family healing, I was able to include my parents in a couple of major foreign trips as well as many local family gatherings. One of my passions in life has been traveling. I learned I could take my program with me. With food in its proper prospective, I learned to be flexible but still keep my abstinence.

My mother died when I was only 34 years old; it was sudden and devastating. I was blessed that we had left nothing unsaid to each other, and I had no regrets. I had been a good son. Like many other things, I went through it with the support of my friends and OA program. I was also able to support my dad, and we became very close.

Little did I know I would lose my dad less than three years later with very little warning. Before then, he was able to be there for my wedding, the birth of my twins, my brother's wedding, and lots of other special times.

With the loss of both parents, I've had trouble always believing in a loving God. I still "act as if" and do my daily OA readings, meditation, and prayer. I know there is some Higher Power; I'm just not sure what it is. But the spirituality I learned through OA works. Even though I'm not a very religious person, with the help of OA, I can take what I like. Being active in our synagogue and sharing traditions with our children has made my life feel richer.

My forties have been about raising my kids, being a husband, balancing work and personal life. I haven't had the luxury of going to five or six meetings a week, giving lots of service, and having lots of time for myself. I had to learn to work the OA program in different ways. With a young family, the balance and moderation that have always been cornerstones of my personal program became even more necessary. I cut down to one or two meetings a week, but I have never stopped attending.

My wife and I have a son who is moderately autistic. He couldn't speak as a toddler, and even at age 14, he is very delayed in speech and abstract thinking. When he was very young, he was hyperactive and unpredictable, and we had to watch him all the time. Again, having the support of the OA program helped my wife and me deal with this issue. When I felt sorry for myself, I could find others who had it worse. I also learned to see the blessing in every situation. Today, even though my son still has far to go, I can appreciate all the progress he has made. By taking care of myself though OA, I've been a better parent to both my children.

As I've aged, one area that has been important is the physical part of my recovery. I found that the same-size meals that once maintained me now cause me to gain weight. This encouraged me to start doing moderate exercise. Since I grew up obese and asthmatic, I didn't want to strain myself. At first, walking a few minutes a day was enough. Then I got an exercise bike. If I did fifteen to twenty minutes every few days, I knew it was better than nothing. A few years later, I joined a gym just so I could vary my routines and not get bored.

Today I actually enjoy moving my body, and I want to feel healthy. I exercise moderately five or six times a week. On the weekends I go hiking or biking with my kids. My family, friends, and coworkers think I'm so healthy, but I am just making amends to my body.

After many years in the same job, I found it had gotten to be more stressful and less rewarding. I prayed and turned it over daily, but for several years I felt stuck. As I was nearing fifty, I could think only of an early retirement.

Over two years ago a new company approached me and wanted

someone with my exact background. With the economy so bad, and having worked thirty years for the same company, I was into fear and didn't want to meet with them. With the help of my OA sponsor and others, I took it one step at a time. After a few months, the decision to leave was easy and clear. I now feel fulfilled and energized in my work again. I am at a company that is aligned with my goals, and I am well respected. This new environment has helped me relook at many things in my life, which is good for my OA program. I am relearning "one day at a time" and how to walk through the fears of change.

Last year I turned 50. I've been both a younger and an older person in OA. When I was new to OA, I thought my life would be boring if I didn't have the excitement of excess food. Well, it has never been boring. I have had many tragedies and sorrows, but because I've been able to go through them without killing myself with food, I have found joy on the other side.

I don't know why or even how, but I've learned that everything happens for a reason. Each day has many things that cause me to feel grateful. Happiness is more about my attitude than my circumstance. The lessons and gifts of OA keep coming as long as I stay grounded in OA.

3

DIFFERENT AGES, SAME PROBLEM

I have been a compulsive eater for as long as I can remember. As a young child, I craved sweets and hid and stole them. I was not overweight until I hit puberty, and even then I only gained 10 to 20 pounds (5 to 9 kg). My self-hate, though, was rampant. I obsessed over what I was eating and how to stay on a diet, never going more than three days without a binge. Food obsession ruled my life and became my nasty little secret.

I joined OA in March 1977. At the time, I was 15 years old and a high school sophomore. I got good grades, was popular, played two musical instruments, had a boyfriend who drove a motorcycle, and had been elected president of my class. I also hated myself and was having suicidal thoughts. I thought if I lost those 20 pounds (9 kg), I wouldn't hate myself anymore.

The only reason I went to OA was that the meeting was within walking distance from my home. I had no idea it was different from other diet clubs. My first meeting was full of women who were older and heavier than I was. Only one person was abstinent, and she was also the only person who had done a Fourth Step. I heard the Twelve Steps read and instinctively knew something was special about them. The people were kind to me, and I decided to come back. I had no intention of staying long, only long enough to lose those 20 pounds (9 kg).

I couldn't lose them. I couldn't get or stay abstinent and started gaining more weight. One night a woman from across town came to speak at a meeting. She was thin and serene. I wanted what she had. I asked her to be my sponsor and started attending meetings across town with her. This was a whole new ball game. The people at these meetings were all working the Steps. They looked at the addiction as a life and death matter. They were recovering. And, unlike my old friends, they didn't coddle me at all. They told me to take the cotton out of my ears and put it in my mouth. They responded to my protests that I was too young and too thin to be a compulsive eater with reminders of all the crazy things I had done with food.

My brilliance and youth did not impress them at all. They did tell me how lucky I was to find this program at such a young age, but I didn't feel that way. To say I was angry is an understatement. Most of them had many good years with food before they found the program. Why couldn't I? As I started dealing with Step One, I got angrier. I didn't want to be different. Couldn't I just lose those pounds, which had now become 30 (14 kg), and leave?

The one thing I've always done right is to keep going to meetings. In fact, despite my anger and resistance, I started going to more meetings. I looked for strong meetings where people took recovery seriously. I began going to other Twelve Step meetings to hear the message that you don't practice your addiction no matter what. I stopped looking at how my youth made me different and looked for things I had in common with other compulsive eaters. As it began to sink in that maybe I was a compulsive eater, I became willing to work the Steps and the Tools. I got a food plan I thought I could live with for the rest of my life. My unwillingness to follow suggestions caused seven sponsors to fire me, but I found a new sponsor and began doing what she told me. By this time, I had been in program almost three years and was afraid a Higher Power was going to zap me dead to show what happens to people who won't follow directions. Luckily, the Higher Power I now believe in is much more loving and patient.

My last binge was January 16, 1980. My sponsor had told me to do a Fourth and Fifth Step, and I got abstinent the week after doing the Fifth Step. Nothing was magical about January 17. On that date, I had a food plan that was comfortable for me; I was going to meetings, doing service, and working the Steps and Tools. I put down the fork after my abstinent meals and didn't pick it back up no matter what. I still do this today.

The miracles I've experienced since getting abstinent are stunning, and my life really is beyond my wildest dreams. I lost the weight and remain thin and healthy at age fifty. I used the Tools and Steps to get through college, graduate school, and professional licensure. I was led to marry a good man, and we'll celebrate our twenty-first wedding anniversary soon. I have three daughters and a healthy relationship with each of them. They have never seen me compulsively overeat.

Ten years ago, I turned over my financial security to my Higher Power and started my own business. I felt led to use unique professional skills to help people who come to me. When I started my business, I was also led to pick up my old electric guitar. Music helps me relieve the stress of work.

Although I am powerless over my level of talent and have many commitments that get in the way, I committed to practice my music fifteen minutes every day. I now play lead guitar in a band that has regular gigs and is a tremendous joy!

I have returned to the faith of my childhood, which is gentle and meaningful. Over the years, I have dealt with deaths, chronic diseases, layoffs, disappointments, and irritations. This program taught me how to deal with all of these without eating compulsively.

Although I believe I can always return to my disease, I also believe long-term recovery is possible, and as long as I do what this program suggests, I can be happy, joyous, and free. That is my wish for all of you.

4

A Mom Who Is Free From Addiction

Pinpointing when my food struggles began is difficult for me. I believe they must have started from birth. In early years, I thought I was always hungry, but my hunger was never satisfied. Now, after many years of working the OA Twelve Step program, I understand food could never fill the hole inside because I suffered from a spiritual hunger.

I grew up surrounded by addiction, as both my parents drank every day. I was the youngest daughter of five, and we all had our separate reactions to life. I ate. My early memories are all about food: chocolate, picnics, movie food, and takeaway nights. I lived for these moments. Money was tight, yet I stole from my parents any coins I could find to spend on sweets. After school I was always ravenous and would empty the cupboards of bread, baking ingredients, cereals, and even foods I disliked. I could not stop.

On our street lived a "dirty old man" that my instincts warned me was unsafe, yet I risked his advances to eat the sweets he bought. Staying away never occurred to me; I had to eat.

When I reached 13, my weight ballooned, and I started a cycle of dieting and bingeing that progressed to swings between anorexia and bulimia. I presented as a troubled teen with eating disorders, but after I stopped that behavior in "happier" years, I still suffered from constant craving and food obsession.

During my youth, I was frequently depressed, which culminated in a suicide attempt at age 16. When my suicide attempt failed, I made a pact with a God I did not believe in that I would choose life no matter what. Many dark years followed. My rock bottom was less dramatic than previous years; it was a sense of blackness so deep that I felt no way out, an intense loneliness and constant feelings of confusion and uselessness.

At age 22, my university studies stalled, my boyfriend left, and I abused my family. Food was my only friend and my worst enemy. I had tried every diet, "loving myself," and "listening to my cravings." I had tried naturopaths and health foods, which were my favorite binge foods. Rather than freedom, I felt fear.

The turning point came at age 27 when my sister Twelve Stepped me into OA. I had witnessed her life of hopeless eating. Within days of starting in OA, she had a sponsor and a plan of eating. I watched her change before my eyes into a loving person who had life between meals. She went to OA meetings, helped newcomers, and was always talking on the phone. Her weight melted away, and a kind, productive individual emerged. For the first time I had hope.

In 1998 I went to my first OA meeting in New Zealand. The Twelve Steps of OA were on the wall, and a group of people talked about freedom from craving and obsession with food. I chose a sponsor, and she told me what she had done to recover. Within days I had my first day off the food. Stopping compulsive eating was a shock, so I reached for a Higher Power. I prayed like my life depended on it, read OA-approved literature, and phoned other OA members. I lived Steps One, Two, and Three.

Slowly, things began to change in all aspects of my life. Then I did Steps Four and Five and began to get honest. Obsession and craving left me around the time I began to be honest. When I told my sponsor my deceptive thoughts, the destructive behaviors stopped. It worked every time, one day at a time, and continues to work many years later.

My work with the Steps began to heal my life. I made amends to family, friends, and others whom I had hurt. Financial amends followed. With every recovery action I took, my hatred for others and myself dissolved. I began to hand over my faults each day. After six months, I started doing OA service and have never stopped. Service makes me feel a part of OA, and I like being useful.

Addiction to food affected every aspect of my life. I was single for fourteen years, seven of those abstinent. After some time in OA recovery, I met my husband and stepson, both of whom I love dearly. My husband and I had a beautiful baby girl together. I feel extremely blessed. When I look into my daughter's eyes, I am grateful that she has a mom who is free from addiction, who is able to love and care for her.

My new family has never seen me binge, eat junk food, gain weight, or plummet into depression. Most important, I am present in their lives. I am grateful that my Higher Power saw fit to extend my recovery to my relationships, community, and children. My loneliness and sense of uselessness has gone.

Every time I walk through the doors of my local meeting, I feel relief. I am now learning about the wider OA Fellowship. I find the OA Twelve Traditions powerful, and when I thought of leaving OA in difficult times, the Traditions helped me to put principles above personalities. I started a meeting in our town, which gave me a chance to grow up in OA. I am learning that my recovery does not involve controlling those around me, whether loved ones or sponsees.

There was little talk of relapse when I came into OA. During a difficult pregnancy, I lost trust with my sponsor, as I was unwilling to put the welfare of my baby into her hands. I began making my own decisions with food like a teenager testing boundaries. This did not work, and my spiritual condition began to suffer. I reached out to a sponsor and became honest once more.

Being honest with an OA member in recovery is the key to Step

One for me. Step One is the Step I am called back to most often. As long as I remember that I am powerless over food and can't do this alone, I can continue to receive this gift of freedom. Thank God for OA.

5

DYING TO LIVE

I am in my fifteenth year of continuous abstinence from food addiction. I came to OA after a spiritual awakening and fourteen years of sobriety in another Twelve Step program. I descended into a horrific food rock bottom, which finally convinced me that compulsive overeating is a progressive, dangerous, and slow-killing disease of mind, body, and spirit. My slide was halted only by seeking help from fellow OA members and taking appropriate actions with the grace of God.

Not everyone has to go as low as I did. Powerlessness over food gradually destroyed my home, career, and ability to drive a car. Eventually I was incarcerated at a mental home for nine months under the diagnosis of a "breakdown." These events were traumatic enough, but the pain in my mind was worse. I kept eating and obsessing against my will, even when I wanted to be abstinent. It was hell on earth.

Why couldn't one miracle—not drinking on a daily basis—solve the problem of a chronic eating disorder? For me, they are separate conditions. Although I didn't know it or want it, I needed to be in the fellowship of other recovering compulsive overeaters and anorexics.

I desparately hoped that self-awareness, therapy, and the other Twelve Step program would help me to iron out the food. But they didn't, and I feared I would die in the food. While in the mental hospital, I could find only one door that offered me hope and a way out: OA.

It's quite shocking to recall that these events happened to me, but the memory helps me stave off thoughts that one day I can eat normally. I never could or will. It also enables me to help others who say, "My food isn't that bad." Mine wasn't in the beginning, but when it was untreated by the OA Principles and program, it destroyed any quality of life for me.

So what happened to help me achieve fifteen years of peace with the food, through the grace of God? It began with one key factor: *I kept going to meetings.* With a damaged right knee, no car, and a walking stick, I got myself to meetings because that was the only place I got any hope—hope that I could be free from the food obsession torturing my mind, hope that life could be different. But I sat there for a long time before the hope started. I couldn't stop bingeing.

Members were a little disturbed by my constant, long sharing on the illness, until finally someone said to me, "Why don't you stop talking and listen? We are abstinent; let's hear about that when you have it." This was painful to hear, but it was true. I was sharing my experience of the illness, but I didn't have any hope or strength to give. I didn't want to do anything to recover, and you cannot transmit something you don't have. Endless talk of my plight wasn't helping them or me. Ours is a program of action to get well. The talk can come later, when we are sane.

The next key factor was asking someone to sponsor me. She said she would, if I truly wanted to be well. I didn't really believe I could be abstinent, but my life was unbearable. I wanted to have all the rewards of recovery without doing anything. I was afraid of going permanently mad or meeting some unpleasant end, but I was stuck.

My next action was to agree to a food plan with my patient, caring sponsor. We gently set times for meals and established which foods were acceptable and which foods were definitely not okay for me. I made a five-minute phone call each morning just to say out loud to another OA member what my plan would be for that one day. It was all I could cope with.

I endured strong cravings and the obsessive desire to cram indiscriminate food into my body. I wanted to give up on my commitment of three meals a day. Knowing I could call my sponsor and other members in the morning, I hung on, prayed, read literature, and walked, waiting for the next OA meeting.

I was physically ill, so I accepted rides, and without planning to, I found myself getting closer to people in recovery. I was known and loved. I later learned to love because it had been given to me unconditionally. It was my responsibility to give it back.

My sole focus for a year became meetings, prayers, phone calls, literature, and most importantly, the simple food plan I shared with my sponsor. This laid down the basis for the first Step, upon which I built a new life and experienced the personality change necessary for recovery. The old me will eat again, so I have to change.

Days became months and months became years. I started attending a home group and doing regular service. Sanity had returned. I had finally been willing to go to any lengths. I worked again, drove a car, acquired an apartment, fell in love, and fell out of love. I supported my family. I was now of use to myself and others. I could (and still do) put out my hand to newcomers and say, "There is a way out. You can live without thinking about food." I had this to offer instead of just sharing about the illness.

On a daily basis, I live in this world as a free woman. I continually apply the OA way of life and have the desire to live humbly under my God's love and direction. It isn't what I have accumulated that makes me happy, but what I can give away to others in this troubled but beautiful world of ours. OA allows me to be a healthy part of that world.

6

THE BOAT STORY

Ecstatic about my purchasing a used sailboat, my wife and 11-year-old daughter joined me in the anticipation of summer days sailing on the lake. I was 40 years old, morbidly obese, and seldom exercised. It had been twenty-plus years since I had sailed. I was also a compulsive overeater, although I didn't know it then.

On a cool February morning, we took the boat out to launch it for the first time. As a strong wind pushed us across the lake, I practiced using all the controls and felt the pleasure of feeling in control. At the end of the lake I turned the boat around, and found that in spite of my efforts, the boat would not go where I wanted it to.

My wife and daughter were laughing, but I was not. When the boat drifted close to shore, I suggested that they walk to the launch ramp. Pushing the boat back out into the lake, I was determined to master the wind, so I could show them who was in control.

Back on the lake, nothing I did produced any movement toward the dock. A young woman in a motorboat, the lake's lifeguard, approached and explained that the lake was about to close. She offered to tow me to the dock and tossed me a line. When I reached over for it, the boat capsized, throwing me into the cold water. Weighing over 350 pounds (159 kg) can have that kind of effect. The lifeguard stopped her motor and offered to help me out of the water. I could not pull myself up into her boat. She wrapped the rope around me and went to the opposite side to balance her boat as she pulled me aboard. I felt frustrated and humiliated. My jeans and work boots were cold and heavy, like my mood.

My wife and daughter wordlessly helped me get the boat on the trailer. I had lost my cell phone, pager, and wallet. These items were easily replaced, though I felt greatly inconvenienced. It never crossed my mind to be grateful that I had survived or that my wife and daughter had not also been thrown into the water.

When summer came, my daughter enrolled in a junior lifeguard program on the lake. I saw this as an opportunity to take her camping and sailing.

On the first day of camp, I dropped her off and timed how long it took to launch the boat. I sailed to the short side of the lake and back. Again, I timed how long it took me to get the boat on the trailer. I was pleased when I picked up my daughter to share the drive home.

The second day I repeated the process of getting her to camp and launching the boat. I was able to sail the boat across the short end of the lake twice before it was time to pick her up.

On the third day, I dropped her off for camp and got the boat in the water with a sense of confidence. As I sailed across the short end of the lake, a strong wind took me up to the end of the lake. I enjoyed the cruise, practicing my sailing skills. I turned the boat and attempted to tack my way back to the launch ramp. The boat turned but went nowhere. I could see the wind rustling the trees by the shore, rippling the water, and tickling my sails, although I was not going anywhere. I was stuck and felt hopeless. It was a disturbingly familiar and uncomfortable place. I thought of my daughter finishing her day at camp and wondering why I wasn't there to pick her up. I imagined her seeing me stuck on the lake and needing to be rescued again. I wondered what that would mean to her.

I had recently begun attending OA meetings and kept hearing a reading that said something like, "We cease praying for our own selfish ends, but may be helped if we pray for others." (*Alcoholics Anonymous*, 4th ed., p. 85) I was moved to say, "God, this is not for me. I believe my daughter needs to have confidence in her father. If it is your will, get me to the launch ramp in time to pick her up. Thank you, God." I was not accustomed to asking God for help with my problems or saying "thank you," let alone thinking about how my actions might affect others. I also did not expect a clear and immediate response.

The wind that had been teasing my sails now engaged them firmly. I sat still, watching in awe as the boat headed straight to the dock. I did not make any attempt to control the boat. I enjoyed a sense that I was being cared for. The boat came right to the dock, and all I had to do was reach out and grab hold.

I wondered about the ways I had been trying to control life, never acknowledging that my Higher Power had a plan for me. I had never considered asking God to help me with my eating and weight. I had only blamed God for making me fat, although I was the one who ate to comfort myself. At OA meetings I saw many people who were recovering from compulsive overeating. Now I knew that all I had to do was ask God to show me the tools and give me the willingness to use them.

In the next eighteen months I lost over 100 pounds (45 kg). I knew my food plan was not perfect, although I abstained from compulsive overeating one day at a time. I had small moments of unexpected joy in this new body I came to live in. Every time I used my credit card, I was asked to show identification. The picture on my driver's license was taken a few days after my experience on the lake, and I no longer looked like that person. Not everyone noticed, but those who did reminded me how much I had changed. When I saw their amazement, it confirmed that a miracle had happened for me on the lake.

It's been over twelve years since that day. Sometimes I ask myself, did that day on the lake really happen? I look at the two driver's licenses I carry, my before-and-after pictures, and I realize that God continues to do for me what I could not do for myself. Today, I am a recovering compulsive overeater. I wrote this story to remind myself to remain like that person on the lake, willing to ask his Higher Power for help.

7

WHO IS MY APPETITE?

I am a 30-year-old Greek woman and recovered bulimic. What a miracle it is to be free to live life, without having to think about food, weight, and body image! I haven't purged in four years, and my food and weight have been healthy and steady for three years.

My bulimia started in adolescence. The pressure to have a flawless body, combined with a sexual awakening and wish for boys to accept me, had a huge impact and led to my first diet at age 15. I lost weight, my period stopped, and the binges started. When my period came back, it was followed by bulimia. The first time I purged was the hardest. I ate so much that my stomach, not being able to digest all the food, hurt and woke me at five a.m. I was sixteen. This cycle of gaining weight, dieting, bingeing, and purging continued until I was nineteen. I knew purging could destroy my insides, so every purge was painful for my body and soul. This is why I would stop purging after a month or less, which of course would lead to weight gain.

As a bulimic, I maintained a normal weight, and others described my body as beautiful, curvy, and feminine. Many confused OA members have asked me why I am in OA. Some fellow members have said that if they had my body, they wouldn't have a problem. How poor of them to think so! Isn't it madness, almost schizophrenic, to live with a problem that exists only in my mind? And if it was so easy, why hadn't I gotten rid of this problem earlier and without help? Why do so many people die from the consequences of bulimia and anorexia?

From ages 19 to 24, I lived purge-free while studying architecture in a Greek city. But purge-free isn't the same as healthy. I changed from a purging to a non-purging bulimic. I continued my dieting and bingeing cycle, followed by yo-yoing weight and yo-yoing self-esteem. I forced myself to go the gym three times a week, not to stay healthy but to lose weight. The former would be healthy; the latter is compulsive for a bulimic.

The yo-yoing devastated me enough to find OA. I wish I could end my story with "I haven't broken my abstinence since," but that was not the case. During my six years in OA, I have learned that what is life-saving for one OA member can kill another. When I joined OA, I was the first bulimic among compulsive overeaters with weight problems. No recovered bulimics were available to sponsor me.

Since I needed recovery and freedom from bulimia, I followed the winning pattern cited in many OA recovery stories: three meals, nothing in between, and no sugar. After living purge-free for five years, this "winning pattern" led me straight to purging after two months of practicing it. I had no one to turn to; all the members were sure this was the way, and we should only try harder until it works out. I tried harder for two years, during which my food plan became stricter and stricter, leaving more and more food categories out. Every time, the pattern failed and led me to a relapse even worse than the last.

I had six relapses in two years. During the last one, I started opening packages of binge foods I was buying while still in the supermarket. My eating disorder was attempting to manifest itself before I had time to change my mind about bingeing.

The turning point for me was working the Steps. The Steps helped me better understand myself and the world around me. They opened my mind as I learned about negative character traits to work Steps Four to Seven. I realized that my emphasis should not be on the food, but on my compulsive control of my weight, which manifested itself in unhealthy ways of eating.

My primary abstinence is not from compulsive food categories but from thoughts like, "You are fat. You are not lovable until you look like this model. You don't deserve to enjoy your food. You are bad, bad, bad!" I also abstain from designating food as "good" and "bad." Taking away the "bad" designation from sweets and allowing them into my normal eating was very hard.

But the hardest thing was to abstain from controlling my body. Learning to listen to my body's signs of hunger and fullness took months of persistence. In those months, my weight increased, which is hard for a bulimic. I had to fight lingering thoughts of dieting to lose the extra pounds. Every time, I said to those thoughts, "No. If it's not now, then it's never!"

Then without my control, without me doing anything, the numbers on the scale started going down. I lost the pounds gained while persisting in listening to my body, and it was my HP's doing! For the first time, I hopped on the scale without knowing if I had lost or gained. In all the years past, my weight loss had been regulated by a strict diet or false abstinence. This time was different. My mind had nothing to do with it whatsoever.

The scale stabilized at the same weight I had been when I first joined OA. The difference was that I hated my weight back then, and now I love it and embrace it. The Step work has made me love myself as I am. Dieting is unnecessary. I am free to eat when I am hungry and stop when I am full. I am free to enjoy sweets when I want them. The most amazing thing is that I don't want them all the time.

My appetite tells me, "Now you need salty, not sweet" or "Now you need carbs, not protein." Who is my appetite? Not me, that's for sure. Let's agree to say it's my Higher Power's voice.

8

Seeking and Finding a Power to Live By

When I was growing up, the only mention of God in my home was preceded by a sneeze. My mother was the only Higher Power I knew. She managed my life, flew into a rage when I displeased her, and praised me effusively when I pleased her. She focused all her energy on making me the person she wanted me to be. Her claim to fame was that she had been voted the prettiest and best-dressed girl in high school. The message I received was that being slim and pretty was the ticket to a happy life.

I married at age eighteen. It was overwhelming but also exciting. I could do whatever I wanted, and I wanted to eat. I was shocked by how much I could eat in one sitting. I would feel shame and remorse at having eaten a whole box of cookies. I vowed never to do it again, and then I did it again the very same day.

Despite some scary overeating episodes, I binged and starved and managed to maintain a normal weight until I became pregnant at age twenty-two. Pregnancy meant I could eat for two. Midway through my first pregnancy, and the two subsequent ones, I took prescription diet pills to stop my alarming weight gains. I still gained

50-plus pounds (23 kg) with each pregnancy. I lost the weight by continuing the pills after my babies were born. The pills were easy to get and doctors never refused my prescription requests.

When I turned thirty, my mother was killed in an automobile accident. The pain of losing her was excruciating, and taking care of my babies without her was unbearable. I threw myself into a frenzy of academic activity and nonstop eating to dull the pain. I went back to school for a master's degree and returned to a full-time teaching position. I earned two more graduate degrees and assumed more responsibility at work.

During this time I could not find doctors who would prescribe diet pills. While taking the pills, I would binge and starve; without them, I binged and dieted with less and less success. I was no longer able to maintain a normal weight.

I found my way into an OA room in 1977 when I was 36. I had two friends who were losing weight in OA, and it was going to be my Diet of the Week. I had a food plan that everyone followed—no sugar or white flour. I came into program needing to lose 20 pounds (9 kg), and I lost 40 pounds (18 kg). I stopped menstruating, and my family told me I looked anorexic. I loved the way I looked and thought they were all jealous. This "diet" lasted for almost two years.

For the next twelve years I had periods of sobriety followed by lapses, relapses, and a final collapse when I left the program for almost two years. During my time away, I added a layer of lies to my compulsive eating by becoming bulimic. If I binged and then got rid of it, everyone would continue to admire me for my slim body. I have learned there is no right way to do the wrong thing. When I crawled back to program in 1989, I was actively bulimic and 40 pounds (18 kg) overweight.

Twelve years after discovering OA, I took Step One. In the past, I had admitted my powerlessness on an intellectual level, but I had never fully accepted it in my heart. The progression of my disease into bulimia finally convinced me of its fatal nature. I was beyond human aid. Bingeing and purging had taken over my life. My obsession with food was a power greater than me. This awareness opened me to the possibility that I could "come to believe" in a power for Good that was greater than me. I felt hope and took Step Two.

I then decided to turn my will (thoughts) and my life (actions) over to a Higher Power (Step Three). Since I still did not have a personal Higher Power, I sought that power by working the rest of the Steps. I had faith that what had worked for so many others could also work for me. Steps Four through Nine allowed me to discern the feelings and actions that were blocking my recovery; admit them to a loving, caring person; become entirely ready to change and grow; and begin practicing the actions that would empower me to treat myself and others with love, acceptance, and respect.

Steps Ten through Twelve now enable me to continue these loving actions on a daily basis. Each day I set aside time to inventory my feelings, quietly reflect on the actions I need to take, and practice the spiritual Principles of the Steps in all my affairs.

I have maintained a normal weight for almost twenty-three years, and I have not had a bulimic episode in over fifteen years. When I make a mistake with my abstinence, I build a bridge to the next abstinent meal. I respond to myself with love and compassion, instead of reacting with self-hatred and more bingeing.

This attitude empowered me to decrease my bulimic episodes until they were extinguished. The same attitude has worked on my binge eating. As I continue living in the Steps and viewing mistakes (painful as they are) as learning opportunities, I release the shame that made me think I was never good enough. For me, recovery is no longer about being thin. It is about treating myself with love and respect. Eating in a healthy way is the most loving thing I do for myself.

I have had a spiritual awakening as *the* result of the Twelve Steps. Prior to program I lived an unconscious life and was not at all aware of "the Great Reality deep down within us" (*Alcoholics Anonymous*, 4th ed., p. 55). My inner Higher Power was covered with negative emotions and excess food. As I followed a plan of eating to stay conscious of what was going into my mouth and used the Steps to stay conscious of what was coming out of my mouth, I found my personal Higher Power. I call that power "Goodness Health and Love." My consciousness of God is consciousness of what is Good in myself, in others, and in the world. When I make time for daily reflection (Step Eleven), I experience that Higher Power as a loving voice that guides me to do the next right thing. I have "tapped an unsuspected inner resource" (*Alcoholics Anonymous*, 4th ed., pp. 567-568), which I now identify with my own conception of a power greater than myself.

I found this program when I was thirty-six and surrendered to the solution when I was forty-eight. I truly believe something I once read, which said there are no failures in this program—only slow successes.

9

SAME DISEASE

W hat are you doing here? You don't need to lose any weight." I feared I would hear that at my first Overeaters Anonymous meeting, and I did.

"I wish I had your disease." You seriously want a complicating factor for compulsive overeating?

"It's all the same disease." Maybe, but the course my disease took required undoing many years of anorexic behavior before I could address compulsive overeating.

My first recollection of body awareness came when I weighed 90 pounds (41 kg) and was a head taller than my younger brothers. Then came puberty and eighth-grade graduation when I lied about my weight. I could not live with a lie, and I lost those 10 pounds (5 kg) in the month before our graduation ceremony. That was the beginning of my struggle with compulsive overeating, interspersed with fasting and undereating, for the next seventeen and a half years.

Having a food obsession does not have to mean eating compulsively. I spent a lot of time cooking or baking, cleaning up after, shopping, feeding others, clipping coupons, and going through recipes. I was always planning how not to eat what others were eating; I did not want to be like the rest of my family with hypertensive heart disease, arthritis, and obesity. Like many overeaters, I struggled with the same 10, 20, or 30 pounds (5, 9, or 14 kg).

In September 1971, I cried out to God, "I can't go on like this. It's the same 10 pounds (5 kg). What used to take nine months or a year to lose and regain now takes ten days of starving and four days to regain. I can't go on like this; it's too hard on my body, too hard on my head." In June 1972, my menses stopped; I was 28 years old. I had meant to lose 10 pounds (5 kg), but then it was another 10 pounds (5 kg) and another 10 pounds (5 kg), seemingly without effort.

Restricting was empowering. I didn't have to take time for sleeping, eating, shaving, or even urinating. I could wear my teenage son's clothes. I shrugged off the comment about "looking yellow." I secretly knew my diet of apples and carrots (when I really had to eat) was impacting my skin color and giving me only enough energy to sit on the kitchen floor.

During a community paper drive, I snatched a medical journal and happened upon an article about anorexia. Now I had a label for what was happening to me. I wrote the author and many months later received a brief acknowledgement of my letter, but no help. On one of my few walks alone, a fleeting thought entered my mind—loneliness. I never felt anything for very long; busyness is a great coping technique. I was the neighborhood nurse and super-mom: the "type E" woman (everything for everybody).

In November 1981, I displaced my tibia. I was anxious about winter coming and limited opportunities for exercise. While attending non-helpful sessions with an eating-disorder counselor, I saw a notice about Overeaters Anonymous. That led me to a contact number in a local newspaper and to my first OA meeting thirty years ago.

I had sought help from a priest, doctor, social worker, and eating-disorder counselor. None could help me. However, in a room full of strangers who were similarly afflicted, I learned I had a disease and that God was interested in something as trivial as my food. Serenity filled the air; prayer started and ended the meeting. Hope was restored. Guilt and shame were released. I had a solution, all in ninety minutes.

I asked the contact person who had accompanied me to the meeting to be my sponsor. I came home and plucked a spiral notebook from the shelf. I started writing about my feelings. God would take care of my weight, so I didn't get on the scales the next morning, or the next, or the next. I had a phone list; I started making calls the next day and the next. God would take care of my food, so I didn't count the pieces of spoon-size shredded cereal.

I read and reread the pamphlet *Before You Take That First Compulsive Bite*. I was back at that meeting the next week. I worked the Steps and used the Tools as though my life depended upon it, because it did. Two months later, fear revealed itself throughout my first inventory. I continued to do mini-inventories on fear every six months until I no longer needed them.

As my home life deteriorated, I had three bouts of anemia along with further weight loss. I decided it was time to quit "waiting for the Lord to do it." I was 107 pounds (49 kg) and 5 feet 8 inches (172 cm) tall. It took me the better part of a year to gain the needed weight by adding a carbohydrate, protein, and fat to my food plan. I didn't realize how thin I was from 1984 to 1985 until I renewed my driver's license in 1987 and actually looked at the photo. I learned that you gain weight the same way you lose it: adopt a sensible plan of eating and stick with it. I have maintained most of that weight, most of the time, for twenty-five years.

My definition of abstinence is sane eating and successful living. In everyday living, it looks likes this: willingness to eat more often, eat more when my weight is down, and increase my use of the Tools when food is calling. Recovery is peace and serenity in my food life, as well as with the people and situations in my life. It is awareness of God in my every breath. Life becomes a prayer.

The OA Fellowship and the Twelve Steps have given me a gift. I treasure the gift of freedom from food obsession.

10

Humility, Gratitude, and Kindness

This morning I found myself alone with several hours of unstructured free time. I chose to go for a hike with my Higher Power and got excited about my plans. Then I chuckled with the realization, "what a difference the Twelve Steps make." Before the program, I would take any opportunity to be alone to eat my binge foods, throw up, then eat more, only to throw up again. Then I would have to replenish the food so no one would find out. My day would end with exhaustion, fear, demoralization, and despair.

At first, eating my binge foods was fun. I was the youngest of four girls in a conservative home with a loving mother and father. Food was very important to us. My childhood was happy even though my weight continued to rise. When I was in second grade, my mother needed to order a customized larger dress for me. This prompted her decision to bring a commercial diet program into the family. Unfortunately, I interpreted the diet program's message as saying that my weight determined whether I was a good girl or not.

Into adulthood, I allowed the numbers on the scale to direct my day. I still remember silly efforts to keep the scale numbers down. I would try standing on one foot, or lean on the wall and let go quickly to see the lowest number and then jump off the scale. It would be a good day if the numbers were "right" and a bad day if I didn't like them. Needless to say, I stayed unhappy with this barometer.

I believed my happiness would come in the future once I finally got to my desired weight. Until then, I would take the bull by the horns and use my willpower to get there. My disease progressed and my world got smaller and smaller. Ninety percent of my thoughts and efforts revolved around my compulsion to eat and obsession with my weight.

When I came to the OA program at 17, my self-esteem was at an all time low. I had drawn imaginary lines based on morality, and then I continuously crossed them. I would say, "I would never steal." But I stole from a broken food vending machine and also from my mom's purse to binge. The disease was consistently turning me into a person I did not want to become. Then I found OA in 1987, and without ever leaving the program, I continue to rise out of those depths of despair.

OA teaches me how to be honest. People in OA meetings share aspects of themselves that I begin to see in myself. OA also teaches me how to love. After twenty-four years in the program, I began to see that self-hatred was my first addiction. I compulsively put myself down, thinking, "You should be thinner. You should have this program down by now. You should be more spirituality fit. You are not good enough. You will never get it."

The Twelve Step program has given me a direct path toward a relationship with God that has solved my eating and weight obsession. This evolving friendship with HP makes me feel good to be alive.

OA meetings are a celebration of life. When I walk into a meeting, I am still in my head. I have many thoughts about what I did earlier that day and what I want to do later in the day. As the meeting format is read, I listen to the words *and* the pauses. The room becomes sacred; there is no hierarchy, no judgment, and an abundance of hope with unconditional love. I always feel much better leaving the meeting than I did when I came.

I have enjoyed continued, imperfect abstinence for over twenty years. I now have a healthy relationship with food because of working the Steps. The Twelve Steps are so good, they need not be done perfectly. I work them to the best of my ability with faith that my efforts are good enough as I grow in the program.

Pride and ingratitude are my biggest character defects. Pride is that hardened part in my mind that needs to be softened by humility and a sense of humor. Making a gratitude list is essential to my daily recovery. I frequently include what I did right each day in my gratitude lists; I believe my focus determines what I become.

Gratitude has become an art form. I have recently been thanking my struggles before they get resolved. Rather than putting my energies into worrying, I affirm what I want (or something better that I don't know yet) and thank God before it happens. As I heard in an OA meeting, "Don't tell God how big your problems are; rather, tell your problems how big your God is." Not all gifts come in pretty packages. In fact, my ugliest moments have been transformed into my greatest assets because they went through the transformative process of the Twelve Steps.

The self-awareness I have acquired in the program is invaluable. I have learned how to discern thoughts of truth from the false thinking of my diseased mind. If I have a thought or idea that energizes me and gives me a sense of connection, it is going to be true. If a thought makes me feel badly about myself or separate from others, it will be false. I am at my best when I am connected to God, others, and myself.

Just as the disease imprisoned me, the OA program continues to expand my life one day at a time. In fact, my life outside the OA rooms has grown to the point where I appreciate being just a member among members. There is no pressure to perform or have the most wisdom in the meeting, and I can contribute just by showing up. Some days, when I don't feel I have anything to say, I quietly pray for the other members to receive inner peace and the gift of abstinence.

My inward journey in OA has been exotic, vast, overwhelming at times, certainly scary, and mysterious. OA provides the love, guidance, security, support, and tools I need to explore within. I learned that my fears vanish once I shine the light of loving truth on them.

Like a treasure hunter, I have found priceless gems beyond my wildest dreams. These gifts become increasingly more dazzling and valuable as I share them with others and keep coming back.

11

VIVID MEMORIES

One of my most vivid memories of this disease happened the summer before eighth grade. I stood in front of the mirror, and all I could think was "fat." I looked down at my stomach and told myself I had to do something about this. The fat had to go. That was the moment food really took over my life.

That summer I went from a 120-pound (54-kg), growing girl to an 88-pound (40-kg) fragment of myself. No matter how much I was able to keep food from entering my mouth, there was nothing to stop it from entering my brain. I thought about food twenty-four hours a day, seven days a week.

It was only a matter of time before my mom took me to a therapist, against my wishes. As this disease has been proven to do, it switched on me. I gained 30 pounds (14 kg) in two months, and my mom allowed me to stop seeing the therapist.

I spent high school at the same weight, but food and body image held the most importance in my life. In my diaries from that time, all I ever said was, "I need to lose weight" or "I need to get him to like me, if only I was thinner." I thought all my problems would be solved if I could just lose weight.

I dabbled with bulimia for a short time in high school, but my mom caught me and confronted me, which scared the living daylights out of me. Exercise became the next best thing to help me maintain my weight.

I lived at home throughout my college career. Over the four and a half year period, my food consumption, along with my physical activity, gradually increased. The more I ate, the more I worked out. My sister and boyfriend were my only friends. I kept the food a secret from everyone. I ate only at night, and I made sure to throw the wrappers away at the gym in the morning.

After my boyfriend broke up with me, the food got really bad. Night after night I would tell myself this binge would satisfy me and I would never do it again. I had to sleep on my back because it hurt too much to sleep on my stomach. Despite the three hours I spent in the gym every day, I began gaining weight.

In November 2004, I reconciled with my boyfriend. I was completely baffled when I could not stop eating. One night, I decided to tell my boyfriend about my problems. I am not sure what came out of my mouth, but I will never forget the two magical words that came out of his mouth: Overeaters Anonymous.

I went to my first meeting in December 2004. In one hour I determined I was a compulsive overeater. For the first time in my life, I did not feel like a square peg trying to fit in a round hole. Two women came up to me and embraced me with love and warmth. Despite my fears and judgments, I know their kindness encouraged me to get to my second meeting.

For a couple of months, I just kept going to meetings and listening. I tried to figure out what abstinence was on my own. I did this by asking others what they ate and then trying to do that. It did not work.

Then someone suggested I get a sponsor. The first thing my sponsor told me was to see a nutritionist. I had my doubts about needing a food plan, but I went anyway. I lied to my sponsor for a couple of months about the binges I was having, but the day I owned up to my behavior was the very day I got abstinent.

For seven months I worked the Steps, getting all the way up to Step Six. What I failed to do was build any sort of fellowship or support around myself. I sat with my problems instead of talking about them, which led me to a one-day binge. The next day my sponsor asked me what my program was lacking, and I knew the answer: fellowship.

That was in November 2005, and I have been abstinent ever since. That one-day binge scared me to death because in those seven months I had already begun to experience the happiness, serenity, and peace others talked about in the rooms. I did not want to give it up that easily, so I started staying afterward at meetings, making three calls a day, and letting others get to know me.

I also started working the Steps over. Step One showed me I am not a normal eater, and that when I try to be, my life is completely unmanageable. Step Two made me teachable. I admitted my old ideas of God were incorrect and changed my concept into an idea that would help me with my compulsive eating and with life. Step Three meant making a commitment. I committed to asking for help with life and not trying to do it alone anymore.

Steps Four and Five, along with Steps Eight and Nine, were the relationship Steps. Four and Five dealt with my relationship to myself. I learned who I was in Step Four and opened my eyes to what I had done. Step Five helped me see it was not so bad and that I could admit it and move on. Steps Eight and Nine dealt with my relationships with others. I had no clue how to be in a healthy relationship. Now I had the chance to make amends and change my behavior. I had the chance to get to know others and let them get to know me.

I continue to work the Steps, using Steps Ten, Eleven, and Twelve on a daily basis. The defects I found in Step Six pop up every now and then. Step Ten helps me to admit when that happens and clear it up as soon as I can. Step Eleven has improved my relationship with God immensely. It is amazing how spending ten minutes a day with God can change the course of my twenty-four hours. And Step Twelve keeps me unselfish. It reminds me there are others out there struggling, others who can experience the same joy I do every day. If I do not share what I have, I will lose it. Step Twelve also reminds me I need to practice what I preach. I can only do that with God.

Today, my most vivid memory of this disease happened during my first year of abstinence. It was the moment I realized what happiness truly felt like. All those years of smiling and pretending were not real. What I got from this program was. That is why today I can say I am a grateful compulsive eater.

12

THE HIKING TRAIL MEETING

I grew up in an alcoholic family. My grandfather was the alcoholic, and my father became very intellectual and out of touch with his feelings. When I was growing up, my mother ruminated food. She got up every night to chew soft, sweet food and then spit it out. As a child, I thought this was normal. We never talked about feelings in our family, and I grew up as an "emotional orphan." I had no tools for dealing with life. I turned inward and became more and more isolated.

After surgery when I was 18, I learned I would never be able to conceive children. I had zero emotional response to this devastating news. I began seeing a therapist, but my real solution for my pain was *food*. I began restricting, starving, overeating, compulsively exercising, bingeing, and purging. Eventually I was bingeing and purging up to fifteen times a day, starving between those times, exercising like a maniac, hating myself, isolating, and living in terror of people.

I thought if I could just find the right food plan, the horrible cravings and obsession would go away. I had part of it right: I needed to avoid the foods and behaviors that caused craving, but that was only the gateway to recovery. The real transformation came from working the Twelve Steps. Otherwise it was just a diet, and that would never help someone like me.

I arrived at the doors of OA on October 10, 1983, at the age of 21, with my life burned to the ground. I was unable to support myself. I was unemployable. I was a wreck physically, emotionally, and spiritually.

By the grace of God, I have been continuously abstinent since April 23, 1987, one day at a time. I am maintaining a 30-pound (14-kg) weight gain. I like to joke that I had to gain 30 pounds (14 kg) just to become thin, meaning I was seriously emaciated when I came to OA.

I have a disease that is physical, mental, and spiritual. I have a physical sensitivity to certain foods. If I eat any at all, it creates a physical craving that I can't control.

Spiritually, I tend to get fearful, resentful, dishonest, and self-ish. This cuts me off from the sunlight of the spirit, and I lose my connection with the only power that enables me not to eat compulsively, one day at a time. If I can stay in fit spiritual condition to the best of my ability each day, God gives me the grace to stay abstinent. I don't feel I need to be perfect in order to stay abstinent. I do need to be willing to go to any lengths to recover through the Twelve Steps, and I need to keep carrying the message of recovery to those who still suffer.

Things didn't get great as soon as I came into OA. I got a Big Book and hope, but I had more eating to do. I spent my first three and a half years in OA in a pattern of relapse and recovery. My last binge was truly epic. I drove an old, junky car from San Francisco to Boston, bingeing on fast food from Colorado onward. Do you know how many fast-food joints there are between Colorado and Boston? I can assure you: It's a lot.

What was different about the day I got abstinent? It was the first time I totally accepted that I have this thing (compulsive overeating), and it is never going away. I truly took the First Step for the first time. I measured out an abstinent breakfast, thinking, "I don't even know why I'm doing this. It's a waste of time." I went to a morning OA meeting, met my sponsor, and accepted her offer of help by going to her house for lunch. She instructed me on what to eat for dinner and told me to go to seven meetings a week, do service, read the Big Book each day, make three calls a day, take quiet time, and call her at 6:45 a.m. each morning with my food written down for the day. I had the willingness born of desperation and did what she said, one day at a time. My life began to blossom.

My second year abstinent, it became clear that I had to learn how to have fun again or I wasn't going to make it. I found a best friend in OA and together we began exploring the world outside our doorstep. Almost every weekend we would pack her tiny car with abstinent food and take off on another adventure. We went bicycle camping, backpacking through the woods, water skiing, snow skiing, and hiking. We visited museums; threw abstinent parties, potlucks, and picnics; stayed up too late dancing; and just generally had fun.

In my third abstinent summer, my OA friend and I quit our jobs to drive across the United States, following our favorite band and going to OA meetings. Later that summer I spent two months backpacking along the Appalachian Trail in the Eastern United States, carrying all my supplies on my back. Every seven to ten days I would stop at a preplanned location to pick up supplies. I had spent months ahead of time dehydrating fruits and vegetables and preparing my food plan. I had friends back home mailing me boxes on the right date to get to the tiny towns' post offices just ahead of me so I could pick them up.

I hiked hundreds of miles over the next several years. These hiking trips were primarily solo, through all kinds of weather, climbing mountain after mountain. I carried a *Lifeline* with me and read it over and over with great joy. I also carried a copy of pages 86-88 from the Big Book. (*Alcoholics Anonymous*, 4th ed.) I cut apart a copy of *For Today* and put the next set of pages in my food boxes, then burned the old ones in the campfire at night. Almost every day

I held a meeting that included me and no one else. I would hold my own hands as I hiked and welcome "everyone" (the committee in my head) to the regular, traveling, hiking trail meeting of Overeaters Anonymous. Whenever possible, I stopped and attended OA meetings along the way.

I have had many adventures in abstinence, based on faith that if I stay abstinent and keep doing this program, things will turn out alright. They may not turn out the way I *want* them to, but things will turn out alright. I survived being accidentally poisoned with cyanide (abstinent), moved 2,000 miles to live the life of a ski bum (abstinent), got a new career and practiced that for seven years in another ski resort, met my husband, got married, gave birth to two children, and now live the daily adventure of parenthood.

It's hard to believe that the person who first came to OA and the person I am today are the same person! The differences are so profound; it's actually a bit surreal. To me, it points to proof of the existence of God.

13

No Longer Held Hostage by Food

As a kid, I was often afraid or bored. I do not know when I started using food to take the edge off my emotions, but I do remember feeling weird about food at a young age. I would scheme to get the last goodie in the box, the biggest piece of whatever, and the lion's share of any food I was supposed to split with my family. Although I was a chubby child, I found that by junior high I could eat whatever I wanted because of my year-round participation in sports. From ages 12 to 19, I was at a healthy, consistent weight for my 5-foot-10-inch frame (178 cm) of between 150 to 155 pounds (68 to 70 kg). However, I was plagued by a skewed body image and failed attempts to eat healthfully.

In young adulthood, my food weirdness crossed the line into addiction. Taking the edge off life required more and more food, and my effort to eliminate all uncomfortable emotions blocked my ability to feel any emotions. I was deeply depressed, spending hours isolated in bed, eating myself sick.

I did many crazy things with food. Once after grocery shopping, I got into my car with all my bags of binge foods, obsessing over the pint of ice cream I had bought to eat on the two mile drive home. After retrieving the ice cream from a sack, I reached for one of the spoons I kept in my glove box. There were none. Shaking, my anxiety grew as I continued to dig through the stuff in the compartment. Suddenly, I freaked out; I scooped out the entire contents of the glove box onto the passenger floorboard, frantically rifling around for something, anything to eat with. Having no luck, I maneuvered a key off my key ring and used it to dig out the ice cream as I precariously drove home.

For a few years, I believed what advertisements, other people, and my insane mind told me: I was unhappy because I was fat. At some point, I realized my real problem was not the food. Something deeper was wrong with me, but I had no idea what or how to fix it. I weighed 335 pounds (152 kg). In the four years since graduating from high school, I had ballooned from a size 9 to a size 30, the largest size available.

I attended my first OA meeting in June 1994 when I was 24 years old. At my second meeting, I was approached by a woman who became my sponsor. In less than a year of working the Steps and following a structured food plan, I lost 160 pounds (73 kg) and had a measure of sanity. My friends and family, who had been baffled by seeing my weight double since high school, were relieved. They believed I was back to "normal" because I was no longer fat. They did not understand what the food did for me: It allayed my fears and boredom, telling me everything would be okay.

After three years, I became too busy to attend meetings or work the program. I went back to using my drug of choice, food, to cope with life. I knew I had a physical allergy, mental obsession, and spiritual malady, but knowing these facts about myself did not keep me out of the food.

The next several years I saw myself reach new bottoms with my food addiction. When I returned to OA, I had gained back the weight I had lost plus a lot more. My new top weight was over 400 pounds (182 kg). Some people may be surprised, but the physical consequences of morbid obesity were not what brought me back to program. The AA Big Book statement, "we had come to believe in the hopelessness and futility of life as we had been living it" (*Alcoholics Anonymous*, 4th ed., p. 25) was my truth. I could not tolerate the spiritual consequences of my overeating any longer.

Recovery this second time has been a journey, an experience made possible by borrowing strength and hope from other members in the Fellowship. I believe that food is not my problem; Food is my knee-jerk solution to life. So, my food plan keeps me sober each day. As I use the Steps to solve difficult situations, my food plan allows me to have a clear head and willing heart to maintain conscious contact with God. I had to practice using the Steps to face life head-on. In doing so, I developed trust in my HP and could let go of food as my solution over time.

I started by abstaining from sugar and attending meetings. I soon began working the Steps with a sponsor as well. As time passed and I consistently prayed for willingness to give up self-will, I began to eat three meals a day with nothing in between. Meals still consisted of second and third helpings, but at least mealtimes had a beginning and an ending.

My sponsor helped me stay focused, one day at a time, on the spiritual solution found in the Steps as I prayed for willingness to further surrender my food issues. Eventually, I became willing to make my meals a single serving. Not-so-healthy food was often piled so high on the plate that parts of it flopped over the sides, but I abstained from filling my plate more than once.

The next part of my process was to become willing to surrender a "God bite," a bite-size portion of food that I left on my plate. The God bite forced me to be conscious of my Higher Power as I ate. I practiced surrendering a God bite at each meal, and I started praying for the willingness to follow a food plan not of my creation. That willingness came nearly eighteen months after my return to OA. As a result, I went through something akin to a detox, and by the grace of God, the mental obsession with food was lifted. I reached a normal weight, having lost more than 220 pounds (100 kg), almost two years later.

Despite the fact that I now look like a "normie," I have to remind myself every day that I will always be addicted to food. Even so, I enjoy many physical, spiritual, and emotional gifts that are the result of living the program. Before coming back to OA, I believed in a Higher Power, but I didn't trust him. Today, I trust that my HP is taking care of me. It is a miracle that I have faced the death of my sister, the beginning and ending of romantic relationships, two cross-country road trips, as well as other difficult life situations, without using food to take the edge off my experiences.

In the course of doing the next right thing, I changed jobs at age 40. After spending years as the fattest person in every setting, I am now a fit, elementary physical education teacher, wearing a size medium instead of the 5XL I once required. I also run 5K and 10K races for the fun of it!

Each day, I carry with me what my food sponsor calls my "hostage food," foods that would allow me to continue my abstinence even if I were to be taken hostage. I enjoy explaining this joke to other people, but I know that every day I must take the actions of someone who is serious about her recovery. OA has given me a new life I never imagined was possible.

14

HE SHARED HIS STRUGGLES WITH ANOTHER MAN

I first came to OA more than nine years ago, but I decided after one meeting it was not for me. My world became smaller and more dysfunctional as I dove deeper into diet programs, fat burners, compulsive overexercising, and purging. I was obsessed with having the perfect body. It took another 60-pound (27-kg) weight gain and five more years of unmanageability around food and relationships before I came to realize I was physically and emotionally sick. After ten years of sobriety in another Twelve Step program, I hated that I could no longer control my eating. I did not feel clean when I binged on certain foods.

My bottom came after my 11 year-old son started emulating my behavior around food. My wife refused to let me drag her and the kids into my disease. I decided to go back to OA, but it took another six weeks of meetings, a major binge over the holidays, and a weight gain up to 260 pounds (118 kg) before I began to attend meetings regularly. My biggest issue with OA meetings at the time was my inability to accept that I could not get one day of clean time. I realized hiding out in other Twelve Step programs was not going to get me abstinent, and what I needed was to be around other overeaters. One thing remained constant: An OA member called me regularly and encouraged me to keep coming back to meetings. I can honestly say this is one of the key reasons I came back to OA.

I heard the word abstinence after my future sponsor kept asking me to read pages 30 and 31 from the Big Book for him. (*Alcoholics Anonymous,* 4th ed.)The task gave me a big resentment, but after a few days, I began to accept I was not like other people. I learned "there is no such thing as making a normal drinker out of an alcoholic" (*Alcoholics Anonymous,* 4th ed., p. 31) and that I was powerless over food. I was blown away when I learned my sponsor had suffered three major heart attacks. He had released more than 100 pounds (45 kg) by committing to a food plan, doing the Twelve Steps, and working OA's Tools every day. For the first time in my life, I felt safe sharing my food and body image struggles with another man.

The next day, January 8, 2009, I wrote out my abstinence list. I made a commitment to my sponsor, my Higher Power, and myself not to eat the foods on my list just for that day. I then made a commitment not to exercise for three weeks to break my exercise bulimia addiction. After four weeks, I had released close to 26 pounds (12 kg), and my life and body began to change in amazing ways. What my sponsor said was true: As long as I attended OA meetings and remained committed to abstinence, the fat would melt away, and I would shrink physically and grow spiritually. Food now tasted different, better. As my sponsor told me, nothing tastes better than the taste of abstinence. I began a daily routine of reading, journaling, speaking to my sponsor and others in the program, attending OA meetings, and doing the Steps. I believe these things have helped keep God in my kitchen.

Today I am grateful to OA for giving me the tools and freedom to make healthy choices around my food. I have been abstinent for more than four years while maintaining a 55-pound (25-kg) weight release. I could not have achieved this without the support of my family, my first sponsor, my current sponsees and stepbrothers, and my friends in recovery.

I remain both committed and indebted to OA for giving me back my life, and to my Higher Power for being patient and loving. In no way am I suggesting that my life is easy today; in fact, I still struggle with my food portions and body image at times. But life is definitely easier and more purposeful because of OA.

15

BINGE FOODS AND DIET BOOKS

From the moment I could open the fridge on my own, I ate compulsively. One of my earliest memories is of standing on tiptoe to reach the cookie jar and ever so carefully lifting the heavy lid so as not to make a sound. I helped myself to several cookies, rearranged the rest to cover my tracks, and then ate them all in secret. Excess food was my ticket to oblivion, and I used the ticket every day. All my allowance went to candy. I could not understand why grown-ups, who had bigger allowances, weren't eating candy all the time.

I went on my first diet when I was 11, and the bingeing and restricting cycle took root quickly. I resented having to eat regular meals. To me, they were wasted calories better consumed bingeing alone in secret. Food was my great solace and reward, the sweetest thing in my life.

Although I was in the merciless clutches of compulsive over-eating, I didn't realize it. I thought I was choosing to overeat and could choose to stop. I was convinced tomorrow would be different. I was never happier than when I had binge food in one bag and a brand new, unread diet book in the other. This allowed me to binge while truly believing it was my last binge because the very next day I would be starting a new diet I would stick to this time.

My bingeing got more and more out of control, and my periods of dieting grew shorter. Unbridled eating was my greatest pleasure. I didn't want to be a "normal eater." I wanted a fast metabolism so I could binge with impunity. I had no interest in eating a few cookies; I only wanted the whole bag and the privacy to binge into oblivion.

I was desperate to be able to eat as much as I wanted without getting fat. I would fantasize about switching bodies with a thin person who worked out. I would take her body, binge uncontrollably, and then give it back a few months later. She would lose all the weight I had gained and give my body back to me so I could binge again. Or I fantasized there was a magic pill I could take that would subtract the calories I ate, so the more I binged, the less I weighed.

As a university student, I had a chance to go away for the summer. I was determined this was going to be the summer I lost weight and kept it off. I wrote a contract to myself, outlining everything at stake and promising, double promising, and triple promising I would remember the devastation of bingeing and never do it again. I still have that letter, smeared with chocolate from my binge the day after I wrote it.

At long last, the realization that I could not stop began to dawn on me. My only hope, to find the right diet and stick to it, had evaporated. Today was hellish and tomorrow would be the same. My doctor told me, if I didn't stop bingeing, I would be crippled in a wheelchair with heart disease by the time I was forty. I turned to him and said, "That information just makes me hate myself more when I binge because I cannot stop."

By the time I crawled into OA, I had already taken my First Step; I had tried everything and wanted to die. Life with excess food was intolerable; life without it was unthinkable. Food had become my master.

Believing in a power greater than myself that could restore me to sanity presented a real challenge. I believed in God, but he was disgusted by my gluttony in a world where people were starving. OA friends suggested to me that I develop a new concept of God, one who could restore me to sanity around food. According to my religious upbringing, creating one's own conception of God was not an option. To do so meant going to hell when I died. But I was so desperate, I was willing to give it a try.

I asked God to forgive me, took out pen and paper, and wrote a description of the kind of Higher Power I would need to take me from food addiction to freedom. I allowed my imagination to soar. I came up with a Higher Power who thought I was amazing, wanted me to have the most gorgeous life, and would send an army of angels to stand between me and the fridge and take away food thoughts whenever I asked. I didn't believe it for one second, but I acted as if I believed. That was enough.

When I came through the doors of OA, I couldn't stop bingeing for seventeen hours; I couldn't stop thinking about food for seventeen minutes. By the grace of OA, I have not compulsively overeaten for over seventeen years. Never once have I asked this imagined Higher Power for help that it has not come.

The spiritual awakening promised as the result of working the Twelve Steps has been the most remarkable experience of my life. I don't know how it works, but it does. In the words of the Big Book, "The central fact of our lives today is the absolute certainty that our Creator has entered into our hearts and lives in a way which is indeed miraculous. He has commenced to accomplish those things for us which we could never do by ourselves" (*Alcoholics Anonymous,* 4th ed., p. 25).

For more than seventeen years, I have enjoyed freedom from compulsion, freedom to enjoy moderate eating, and the joy of carrying the message of OA. The gorgeous life of my imagining has become reality. I recently turned 40, and instead of being confined to a wheelchair, I gave birth to a healthy baby girl. Instead of heart disease, my heart is bursting with joy with the daily reminder of the depth and wonder of the grace of God.

Thank you, Overeaters Anonymous!

16

The Turning Point Came

I am a recovering compulsive over- and undereater who grew up in a loving but imperfect family. I felt pressured by my mother's expectations and had no voice in the family. I presented as a good girl, but I learned to be sneaky to get my way.

I grew up eating healthy and my weight was never a problem until my body started to change. It did not change the way I wanted it to! My breasts were small and my hips and thighs were disproportionately large. I remember every comment others made about my body, and how inadequate I felt.

Trying to fit in, I started to exercise and limit my eating. I lost some weight, but my life didn't change. Perhaps my disappointment that "thin is not well" opened the door to comforting myself with excess food.

My eating was somewhat controlled while I lived at home, although I binged while babysitting and pilfered sweet treats at the store where I worked. Once I was in college, my cycles of over- and undereating escalated. I began trying to control my weight by abusing laxatives, smoking in secret, and avoiding social occasions involving food. I didn't realize it at the time, but these behaviors also removed me from the social situations where I felt so inadequate. I felt temporarily better about myself, but my world got smaller.

I felt it was most important for my outside to pass as normal and for others not to see the mess that was inside. As long as my weight was somewhat controlled, I justified my bizarre habits, which included starving all day and eating all night, obsessing with the scale, overexercising, and other bulimic behaviors.

Trying desperately to fit in, I turned to alcohol and my life quickly spun out of control. I got sober in a Twelve Step program, but I still turned to food to deal with the unpleasant feelings and difficult situations I confronted in the real world. My focus on food, weight, exercise, and body image kept me from looking under the surface to confront the key issues that fueled my addictive nature.

One day, my Higher Power let me know that I didn't get sober just to die inside from another disease. I went to OA that night and put down what I call obvious sugar. I went regularly, but I tried to get well by passively attending meetings without connecting with people or doing any work.

A turning point came when I contracted a serious illness that meant I had to avoid fatty foods, and for the first time ever, I experienced intense cravings for fatty foods. Each time I gave in, I became violently ill, until I finally got the message that my disease was bigger than just being a sugar addict. I saw that my disease would continue to morph into other harmful foods and food behaviors— and even other addictions—if I didn't start to take my program very seriously. I identified the foods and food behaviors that didn't work for me, and every day I asked for the willingness to stay away from them. I started using the Tools and began to work the Steps again, this time from an OA perspective.

I wrote my food history in gory detail, and that helped me to stop minimizing the impact of this disease. It was clear that, no matter what I weighed, I believed I was not good enough, and I had lost an inordinate amount of time consumed by food obsession. I knew that my loving HP would not want me to hurt myself any more, and

I turned to that power for daily help.

My Step work focused on Steps Six and Seven, which I had previously glossed over, probably because I could indulge certain defects and still not pick up a drink. But to eat in a healthy way every day, I had to let go of more of my shortcomings. Otherwise, I would continue to behave badly and turn to the food for escape.

Anger and my critical, controlling nature were the most challenging defects for me. Through self-will I tried to be a "good girl," but the frustration and anger built and came out in hurtful ways. I began to hate myself for these defects and lost sight of the fact that this was only one aspect of who I was. Working Steps Six and Seven helped me see what anger did both for me and to me. I learned that, whatever benefit a defect gave me, there was a healthy program way to achieve that same benefit. I learned to speak up for myself instead of burying my feelings. Now, when these defects inevitably return, I recognize them early on and work my program to express myself in a healthy way.

My food and the way I work this program have evolved during my years in OA. Every day, I still need to take quiet time in the morning to talk to my HP and listen for guidance. I also plan my three meals and optional snacks and make sure they fit around the activities of my day. I do spot-check Tenth Steps frequently and listen for the voice of my disease. When it tells me to eat inappropriately, I look closer to see what is really bothering me so I can deal with the actual problem. When my disease speaks more subtly through repetitive negative thoughts, I consciously call on the voice of my recovery through prayer or picking up a Tool. If I indulge in diseased thoughts, I will inevitably betray myself again through bad behavior and eventually the food.

I have learned more from sponsoring than from any other Tool. One of my first sponsees taught me to be grateful for a body that works, and this prayer has helped to release me from my most severe body image issues. Another sponsee helped me see that "half measures" may avail me something, but that we all deserve the threefold recovery we can receive if we make recovery our priority.

Sponsoring has also helped me to be much kinder to other people in and out of the rooms, as well as to myself. I have learned valuable lessons from every person I have worked with, and I am grateful I had the courage to say yes to this service.

When I came into OA, I wanted to develop a healthy relationship with food. Only after my food was in its place could I see that I needed healthy relationships with people instead. Now, I have meaningful relationships with my Higher Power, the people in my life, and myself. I lead a full life thanks to this program.

17

Don't Let Me Waste an Iota

I'm an orthodox Jew living in Israel, and I'm a recovering compulsive overeater. I have been abstinent for almost eleven years and have been maintaining a 165-pound (75-kg) weight loss.

I am by nature one of those people who are clueless about how to live life. For a long time I felt that God put me here but neglected to give me an instruction manual on how to live. It's also clear to me that I am wired to eat. Inhaling enormous quantities of food was the best way I could cope with the pain of living.

My elementary, junior high, and high school years were all unmanageable. In the beginning I felt only that I didn't fit in; by the end I was a complete outsider. Eventually I managed to get kicked out of high school (but with a diploma) about six weeks before the end of twelfth grade.

The following year I attended a religious, post–high school program. I lasted seven months before I was asked to leave. I then tried another religious school for two months. At that point it was clear to me that I did not belong in religious school, and I started a series of jobs. Each of those lasted a month or so until I was fired.

I also tried enrolling in a local state college. Halfway through the first semester I stopped going to class; my grades for that semester were straight Fs.

My parents sent me to a psychologist, and he unofficially diagnosed me as being unable to feel my feelings. With his help I was able to get a job and hold it for two years; after that, I was able to go back to college and complete my degree.

In the meantime, I used food to get through each day. Food was magic; it numbed me and gave me the ability to carry on. I never felt full, so I learned to stop eating when the package was gone. It goes without saying that I preferred family-size packages.

I got married a year before I finished college and got my first real job at the beginning of my last semester in school. Then I began a fifteen-year stretch of isolating and eating to get through each day. By the end of that era, I started my typical day by eating a large meal on the one-hour drive to work, plus one or two stops at convenience stores. At work I ate to get through scary tasks. After work I stopped for food as I drove home, and I ended each day with an enormous binge I called supper.

Life finally got unbearable in the fall of 1999, and I started looking for the ultimate fix. In December I went to my first OA meeting, and I met people who saw food the way I did. As I continued in OA, I encountered people who succeeded at abstinence and serenity. After about six months I got a sponsor. As my involvement in OA grew, I listened to countless speaker tapes, I lost the excess weight, and my soul began to heal.

The first lesson I learned was how to eat safely. I found that I needed to weigh and measure my food to keep from fooling myself about quantities. For the first few years I also found it extremely helpful to pre-pack my food, so whenever the clock struck "eat," I would not be foraging in the kitchen. I still pre-pack my food whenever I feel the slightest risk (holiday meals, family events, or when I'm an invited guest).

I also learned in program that I am enough. When a sports team manager assembles a team, he or she looks to combine a number of players into a single unit. The manager does not expect a group of perfect players who play perfectly every time; rather, the manager collects individuals with different strengths who will complement the team as a whole. The manager wants every player's unique touch when that touch is especially needed.

I learned that God puts me in places where he wants my unique touch. He does not want me to perform the task perfectly; rather, he wants my contribution to affect the situation in my own special way.

My favorite thing about the program is that I have learned to live with integrity. To me this meant learning to ask God for help each day, to direct me to his will for me, and to keep me from trampling other people with my own self-will. It meant learning to contribute what God has given me to offer, without looking for what I could gain. It also meant learning to perform regular self-examinations, to become aware of my behavior, and to fix what I have spiritually soiled.

After a year and a half in program, I went overseas to visit my parents. For the first time I was able to recognize that they were pushing my buttons. Miraculously, it was okay. I remember waiting at a bus stop a week into the visit and suddenly realizing that the hole inside me had closed.

Sayings I like to keep in mind are "esteem-able acts bring self-esteem" and the Navajo expression, "If I don't turn around now, I might end up where I'm heading." When I remember those two principles, my day goes a lot better.

As a big part of my daily program, I ask God to remove my defects of character and to have me be the best I can be. For my daily defects portion, I have divided my Step Seven defect list into five pieces, one each for Sunday through Thursday: selfish, dishonest, self-seeking, fear, and wired-this-way. I also write a summary of my outstanding amends on Friday, and I write a list of components that comprise my Plan of Living on Saturday. For my be-the-best-I-can-be portion, I make a list of things I feel I need to ask for help with every day.

I close each morning's prayer with surrender and gratitude:

"God, I cannot carry out (or even know) your vision for me and my life. Please God, take me and lead me to realize your vision for me. God, I am scared that my life will be a wasted opportunity; please, please, don't let that happen.

"God, please help me recognize that everyone and everything you put in my life today is absolutely the best thing that could touch my life. And most importantly, please don't let me waste an iota."

18

KEEP COMING BACK FOR THE MIRACLES

At age 28, I started bingeing and purging. I had failed at everything in my life, and I gave up. But how did all that get started?

My first twenty-two years looked pretty good from the outside. I had a good family and a middle-class upbringing. Both my parents were kind and caring people, as are my brother and sister. I must have been switched at birth, because no one else in my family has this disease. However, I never quite fit in anywhere until OA. I tried, but I was socially off and very shy. As a minister's family, we moved a lot, and that set me apart. On top of that, I realized I am a lesbian and felt isolated even more because of my fear of being discovered.

I graduated from a university in the south with a master's degree in health and physical education. (Note that my health knowledge did not help me overcome my eating disorder.) I failed at relationships and jobs for several years until I gave up and turned to food. When I started gaining weight, I looked for a solution and began throwing up. I am lucky that I didn't pop my eardrums or hemorrhage from the projectile vomiting. I sincerely hope no one reading this story decides to try bulimia, because it was life threatening for me.

Bulimia took over my life from then on. I would get up in the morning, eat until I was stuffed, and throw it all up. Then I cleaned up, got dressed, and went to work. (By then I had a job to support my eating habits.) I ate nothing until after work, when I went to the store. I changed stores every day so no one would notice how much I bought. I got enough food to feed a big family (of course, it was only me) and put it in the trunk of my car. After dark I carried it into my house. When I finished my six-to-eight bouts of bingeing and purging every day, I carried the garbage out to the dumpster (I got to be good friends with the neighborhood cats.) I continued this pattern for fifteen years.

My bulimia caused many problems: dehydration and hospitalizations; dental problems and loss of teeth; loss of muscle (I loved to play sports but couldn't do it); damage to my esophagus; a black mark on the side of my forehead where I held it when I threw up; no menstrual cycle for ten years; jaw problems; acid reflux and stomach problems. I had no friends and did nothing away from home except work. I was very lonely because I hid and ate.

The food came before people, family, or friends. My best illustration of this came from the night when I was bingeing and my landlady upstairs started screaming for help. I did not go to her aid at once but went to throw up first. When I was through purging, I went upstairs to see what was going on. Her ex-husband had been beating her and left when I got there. Sadly, my disease was more important than her safety. I was very ashamed.

During my years of overeating and purging, my family of origin encouraged me to get help. With their financial assistance, I went to four treatment centers and three halfway houses. I did not get recovery from the treatment centers, but they offered lots of craft activities. I made all my Christmas presents one year, and I still have my $20,000 Santa Claus ceramic boot to show for it. The treatment centers kept me alive, but I still binged and purged.

I hit bottom when I lost my job in 1989. I had nothing left, and

I knew I was killing myself. I learned about a recovery residence in a large city and went there in 1990. I had to go to OA meetings every day, and that is what worked for me. I heard your stories of hope and about a solution that worked. After two years in recovery, I suggested to my parents that I might return home to help them out. Without hesitation, they both said, "Oh, no, stay where you are doing well." I am grateful to my HP that they were able to see me in recovery and I got to thank them for all their help before they died.

I was teachable when I got to OA, and when people said to get a sponsor, I got three. I met with my sponsors every week to study the Big Book and the OA *Twelve and Twelve* and to work the Steps. I got up early each morning to read, pray, and meditate for an hour. From an OA member's suggestion, I put my shoes under the bed so I would have to get down on my knees to pray. I wrote down my food and gave it to someone. I planned my meals each week and grocery shopped with someone else.

I went to a meeting and called one of my sponsors every day. I hung out with recovering people and seldom ate alone. After a year of recovery, I started doing extra service. I led Step studies or Big Book studies at two treatment centers. My recovery life, OA service, and time with OA friends gave new meaning to my life. In 1996 I went back to school for a new career in a health service field. I worked helping others for twelve years until I recently retired in 2011.

To maintain my recovery, I still do OA service, sponsor people, go to a lot of meetings (I love OA people), call my sponsor, work the Steps, follow my food plan, pray, meditate, and study the literature. By the grace of HP and working my OA program, I have been abstinent more than twenty-one years.

Recovery has not all been easy, however. In 1990 I was diagnosed with chronic lung disease. My physical health deteriorated even as my OA recovery developed. Although I ate healthy food and exercised as much as I could, my lungs got worse. After ten years of recovery coupled with declining health, I received a lung transplant —another miracle gift of life. A wonderful aside to this story is that

I was able to play sports again after my transplant. I was 60 years old and playing softball, thanks to HP, OA recovery, and my organ donor and his family.

I have a wonderful, supportive, loving partner of sixteen years and have been adopted by her lovely family. My brother and sister trust me around their food and actually like me. I am truly blessed and enjoy my life of recovery, play, service, and freedom from food. I hope I can give back in the same way I have received. Thanks, OA!

19

THRIVING AFTER RELAPSE

By the grace of God, I am a relapse survivor and becoming a thriver!

My first memories are of cinnamon toast with sugar and a list of sweets as varied as the letters of the alphabet. My parents were active in the Civil Rights Movement. As a little girl I met now-famous people, but meeting them is fused in my memory with what I ate.

I was an average-sized child. My weight gain occurred at puberty when I ballooned past an average weight. Overeating was central to my high school experience. The only time I lost weight was when I prepared to go to college. I brown-knuckled not eating by dividing the calendar days into four blocks. If I ate the food on my diet during a block of time, I blacked it out. I willed myself through many blacked-out months before I made it to college looking normal, but not goal weight.

I loved college and inched into the upper range of a "normal" weight. I learned being nearly normal-sized didn't stop me from having my heart broken during college and beyond. Each time led to a weight gain.

I graduated and joined the workforce. Bam! My eating and weight burst through dress sizes. I was open to the invitation I received from my boss, another African-American woman, to join OA. OA made it clear that I wasn't going to recover without a Higher Power. I knew *something* was greater than me.

Every day after work, a convenience store at the base of a seventh-floor building loomed as tall as the building in my mind. My desire for specific junk food and a craving in my body would rise up to meet it. I couldn't walk by without stopping in.

I met my Higher Power when I walked through Step One in front of this store. I accepted my powerlessness: "If you are real, you will have to help me get past this store. I just can't do it alone." I started walking, looking straight ahead. As I walked beyond the store, I felt a freedom I had never felt before. This was my spiritual awakening that the God of my understanding cared and would help me, if sought.

I went to meetings, found my sponsor, and began to practice the program. I was taking Step One; I eagerly believed I could be restored to sanity; and I turned my life and my will over to the care of God. My conscious contact with God, practicing the Steps, being sponsored, and sponsoring others were critical to remaining abstinent for the last five of my ten years in OA. Steps Four through Nine resulted in my making amends to my father, with whom I had a strained relationship, and my sister, whom I had treated poorly when we were growing up. I became a sponsor and had the honor of hearing several Fourth Steps.

I joined a church and accepted the God of my understanding on a deeper level; however, I was ignorant. When I heard God was the healer, I thought I was cured. I walked out of the rooms and stopped practicing the program.

I was in relapse for eight years after a ten-year period of improvement in the rooms. In relapse, I didn't pick up sugar for the first four years. I slowly started gaining weight, but after I took that first compulsive bite, I regained the 30 pounds (14 kg) I had lost and gained 30 pounds (14 kg) more.

The disease is progressive. I used to eat three doughnuts in one sitting; now I was eating eight. Where I used to eat two pints of ice cream, I now polished off three, plus complete pound cakes and cans of icing.

I heard the first whisper to return to OA from a question in a sermon. "What are your idols? Money? Food?" I didn't hear the rest of the sermon. I was worshipping food because I placed it before God. I kept eating into a size 22.

It took six months for me to hear the next message. I was in a prayer meeting, and a young man from another Twelve Step program confirmed what I was experiencing with food: He had difficulty reaching God when he was using drugs. After the meeting I told him I had been in OA. He said two words, "Go back."

My Higher Power gently encouraged me with one more message. I called the general OA phone line to find a meeting. I recognized the person who answered, and she welcomed me home.

I hit bottom, and the work began. My first time in program, I gradually gave up sugar and ate smaller portions over time. Although I believed I was powerless, I thought I was helping God with my recovery.

During relapse I had experienced *complete* powerlessness and the totality of God's grace. When I returned to OA, my father was diagnosed with prostate cancer, and an old boyfriend re-entered my life and proposed. I held onto practicing the Twelve Steps and the Tools of the program, just as someone who grabs a rope from a helicopter when the roof of the house is about to give way to flood waters.

I learned that God offered me the gift of abstinence at all times. It was true grace; I couldn't earn it. I had to pray for the willingness to ask God to help me. And I have accepted the gift one day at a time for over eleven years.

My first sponsor relapsed and left the program. My next sponsor was a longtimer from another state. She taught me that I needed to use the HOW of the program daily. Was I being Honest? Open-minded? Willing? She taught me how to practice the Steps and use all the Tools.

This time, I accepted that my body had an allergy to sugar and that my craving was insatiable. I had to take a leap of faith and believe the nutritionist knew what she was doing when she gave me my specially designed food plan. I began to weigh and measure my food. I fought negativity by using my faith's literature and the AA and OA literature partnering in the battle.

My practice of the program revealed that it wouldn't be wise to marry my former boyfriend. I became a sponsor on the day I would have married. Surrounded by loving members of OA, I chose to continue to walk in progressive recovery instead of regressive relapse.

I joined our intergroup after years of attending meetings, accepting that I had a responsibility to the Fellowship beyond the meetings I attend. My Higher Power's grace meets and directs me every time I take any of Twelve Steps into progressive recovery. What joy! God is directing me into my purpose, and I was sent back to OA to serve.

My boss Twelve Stepping me into OA was one of my greatest gifts. My Higher Power bringing me back to OA showed he can love everyone back into the rooms, no matter how long they have been away. This is a gift I want to share with every struggling compulsive eater, no matter what their race.

Welcome back. Welcome home. There is a loving place for you in the rooms of Overeaters Anonymous.

20

FOOD FOR THOUGHT

After four decades of relapsing from diet after diet, I have maintained my abstinence from compulsive overeating for over two years now. I consider this a miracle, and I attribute it to working this program as a three-legged stool like OA literature teaches us. Working the spiritual, emotional, and physical aspects of this program is what makes it different from the endless assortment of diets that I relapsed from again and again.

I work the physical leg of my program by following a definition of abstinence, as well as a food plan, that sets me up for success. I have identified my trigger foods and avoid them. I engage in exercise I enjoy almost every day.

I work the spiritual leg of the program by letting go of my doubts about what God may or may not be and praying anyway. A prayer creates space between craving and overeating, so I can make a new choice. I watch how my thoughts change afterward, and I open my heart to guidance in all the ways it might be conveyed. I take a STOP (a Spiritual Time Out Please) any time of day when I need to get more calm and centered because I am less compulsive when I am calm.

I work the emotional leg of the program by tuning in deeper to my feelings instead of avoiding them with food. I use my Step work to grow more aware of my emotional triggers for overeating.

I trace those triggers back to my childhood (Step Four) when I first learned how to bury my emotional reactions to troublesome events. And I use the subsequent Steps to bring those buried emotions into the light, reinterpret those early experiences, and choose new responses.

But there is more to my recovery. I recently discovered there is also a mental or cognitive aspect to this program that has been absolutely critical to my recovery. How I *think* about food and eating has been a key component of my success, and I have come to think of it as the fourth leg of my recovery stool. As a recovery friend said, "I can't help the thoughts that pop into my head. But after that, it's up to me." Recovery has taught me that I have control over my thoughts; my thoughts do not control me. To gain that control, however, I had to honestly examine my thoughts and attitudes about food and eating. Most of them, I found, were filled with illusions and denial.

The first illusion I uncovered was thinking of food as a comfort. How could I label something comforting if it made me miserable after the first pleasurable sensation? By definition, comfort should be enduring, calming, and relaxing, not something that evokes guilt, shame, and misery. The first thing I did in program was to draw up a list of things that truly give me longlasting comfort. I turn to that list when I have a craving, and I incorporate those things into my life as often as possible.

Another damaging illusion was my attitude about abstinence. At first I associated abstinence with restriction and deprivation, like a diet. I thought of eating whatever I wanted as abundance. I had that backwards! Overeating was the source of most of the scarcity in my life: scarcity of energy, health, peace, pride, and self-esteem. Abstinence has been the root of the abundance I now have: increased energy, growing self-esteem, pride I feel when I go to bed at night, pain-free living, choices I now have at the clothing store, good health, and peace I live with now that the war is over. Abstinence, not limitless food, brought these riches.

Another change I needed for recovery was to think more consciously about what I eat, rather than eating distractedly. Now I look at my plate before I eat and say to myself, "This is my meal. I may want more after I'm done because that is the nature of my disease, but I won't act on that. When I'm done, I'll get up from the table and do something else." And then I look at my food and consciously enjoy every bite, becoming aware of the feeling of fullness as I eat.

I have learned to view recovery as a process, not an event. A diet has a beginning, middle, and end. Recovery is a one-day-at-a-time way of life. When I embraced that idea, I stopped watching the scale and began living a life that made me feel confident, connected to others, and serene—all feelings that counteract compulsiveness.

I'm also learning to think about recovery in tiny increments like baby steps. Looking too far ahead overwhelmed me. Now when I have a craving, I ask my Higher Power for the help, strength, and courage to do the next right thing, whether that's to walk the dog, wash the dishes, or weed the garden. In tough times, I work my program one *moment* at a time, not one day at a time. If I become overwhelmed, I ask myself, "Can I just do this today?" and I let the future stay there.

I now choose what I focus my thoughts on: Do I spend more time thinking about what I can't eat and how much I miss it, or do I change my focus to what I can eat, maybe looking up new recipes, learning about new spices, and more.? Do I "change the channel" of my thoughts as I do when a food commercial comes on TV, or do I encourage dangerous thoughts that threaten my abstinence? I make these powerful choices many times a day. If I'm aware, I can choose differently.

I also choose not to focus on what I didn't do perfectly in a given day. My yoga teacher said, "What we think about and talk to ourselves about all day is what we manifest more of in our lives." I ask myself every night, "What did I do right today?" If I end my day by focusing on any success, however small, abstinent or not, I am more likely to build on that success tomorrow.

I look, too, at my general attitude about life. Do I have an attitude of gratitude and hope? I can choose whether to focus my thoughts on what is going wrong in my life or what is going right. Almost every day has some of both. Focusing on gratitude and hope gives me a sense of balance and peace and, in that state of mind, I feel much less compulsive.

What are my thoughts about food and eating today? Are they based in the illusions of my disease or in the reality of recovery? Do they enhance my feelings of success? Do they give me hope and gratitude? If not, why not choose other thoughts? It's in my power; something I can do any time, any day.

That's food for thought.

21

TOOLS AT MY FEET

I am a compulsive overeater from Christchurch, New Zealand. I first went to an OA meeting twenty-five years ago. I'd like to say I've been sober ever since, but there was a seventeen year lag between attending my first OA meeting and admitting my complete defeat.

Thirteen of those long, miserable years were spent in the rooms of another Twelve Step program. If that's not insanity, I don't know what is.

All that time, I put up a false front. I had a good job and was heavily involved in sports. I had a wife and two kids I loved, a house and a car, but food always came first. I clamped a smile on my fat face, but I was crying and dying inside.

I always knew there was a solution in OA. I saw it in a couple of people at my very first meeting. They were free of the fear, guilt, shame, anger, and humiliation, which had always accompanied my eating. They told me if I wanted to get well I'd have to give up eating, drinking, and drugging. They offered me an answer, but I flung it back in their faces. For years I went in and out of OA's doors, insisting I wanted to do it my way.

My eating was no different than theirs. I believe I was born an addict. I remember always having the obsession to eat and the craving for more. I stole food, ate burned or soiled food, and scrounged for food in rubbish bins. I screamed at the staff in a fried chicken joint because they'd run out of chicken. Once I started eating I couldn't stop; I was powerless over the craving.

When I was 12 years old, a classmate collapsed with a ruptured spleen. He'd barely hit the floor before I was plotting to steal his lunch. I furtively got in line and mumbled his name. I cradled his bag of sausages and chips to my chest like a baby. Yet, for so long, I kidded myself that "my case is different." I was a man for a start. I can't recall any men at my first OA meeting. There still aren't a lot here, but I no longer believe this is a "woman's problem."

For years I deluded myself that I could use another Twelve Step program as a one-stop shop for all addiction ills. That never worked either. I can stay sober only alongside other compulsive overeaters.

This is certainly a fatal, progressive disease. I was 25 when I first came to OA. I was 42 when I started to get well. Near the end, I was separated from my wife and kids and was living just to eat. Every day I woke up, determined to "beat it." Within an hour I'd be eating, and the sordid cycle would start again. I fought the urge to drive into the base of a bridge, so I could break a leg and get some time in a hospital, some respite from my head.

So, what changed for me? The two most expensive cans of cola in the world were a catalyst, but the real impetus came from my Higher Power.

I was working overseas and got ensnared in a bar scam in Paris. A French woman I'd met on the Champs-Élysées drank two bottles of champagne. This so-called sober alcoholic slugged two cans of cola and choked on a bill for around $1,200.

Back in my hotel, having had to explain why I'd charged it to my company credit card, I knew my actions were not those of a sober man. My Higher Power sent me the message: I was as powerless over food as I was over booze.

I came back to Christchurch and went to every OA meeting I could. But I still had the obsession for some months. I badgered another new member for a food plan and adopted her breakfast and lunch. Yet all day, my head was consumed with what I would eat for my "free choice dinner."

My recovery started when I did the one thing I'd never done in OA before—ask for help. I remember my sponsor asking if I was entirely ready to give up the food. I said, "I can't say one hundred percent, but I think I might be." Something shifted then.

When I called her the next day for a food plan, the fight I'd had all my life had somehow gone. I'd finally let go of my old ideas.

I haven't had to eat since. After accepting I was a newcomer, I came to understand the answer wasn't in the food plan. I set out to work the Steps of recovery beginning with Step One. I did my first real, searching moral inventory.

It was a shock to find I had harmed many people, and it was humbling to make direct amends to the people I'd insulted and assaulted many years before.

Almost nine years on, I'm grateful that the obsession to eat has been removed. I try to show my gratitude by following the example set by my sponsor and many others in pulling my weight (once a Herculean task) in doing service. I strive to live my amends by being a better dad, grandfather, son, brother, friend, and worker.

The Big Book contains four words that pretty much sum up any (self-induced) problem I have today: "He begins to think" (*Alcoholics Anonymous*, 4th ed., p. 61). I still have one of those magic, magnifying minds that focuses more on what I don't have than what I do have. My sponsor still regularly reminds me that, with a hairstyle like mine, if I keep staring at my navel, I'm going to get sunstroke.

A slow learner, I've discovered there are no Big Book chapters titled "Into Thinking" or "Into Feeling," just "There Is A Solution," "How It Works," and "Into Action."

I'm still a compulsive overeater; I'm not cured. But no matter what happens in my life, good or bad, I don't have to eat, one day at a time. I'm very grateful that God has removed the obsession.

I try to express my gratitude by carrying this message to still-suffering compulsive eaters and to others, like me, who struggled in other Twelve Step fellowships. It took me so long to pick up the set of spiritual tools laid at my feet. Now, it's a privilege to give them away.

22

OA IN GUADALAJARA AND AJIJIC, MEXICO

THIS IS THE STORY OF OVEREATERS ANONYMOUS IN
GUADALAJARA, THE SECOND LARGEST CITY IN THE STATE
OF JALISCO, MEXICO, AND ITS SISTER MEETINGS IN AJIJIC,
A FISHING VILLAGE LOCATED ON LAGO CHAPALA,
MEXICO'S LARGEST FRESHWATER LAKE.

M y recovery started when I attended my first OA meeting in Plano, Texas, in 1981. In 1989 I moved to Oklahoma, then retired in 1997, and moved to Mexico. I knew there were Twelve Step meetings in my area but no OA meetings. After two years with just emails and calls to my sponsor, I started a weekly OA meeting. I registered the meeting with the World Service Office, placed flyers on bulletin boards in two small towns, and put ads in the local papers. We held the first meeting in November 1999, with six women in attendance.

This is a vacation and retirement community, and people come and go. We have quite a few part-time residents from the United States. These snowbirds are in OA in other parts of the US and Canada, which brings new insights to our meetings. Originally we had only one meeting a week until a member insisted on having two meetings; the second meeting starting in 2001. Attendance ranged from three to six OA members, with the largest attendance being twelve.

Many times I was the only one at meetings. I kept asking my HP for guidance and to send people if the meetings were to continue. Doing this service has kept me abstinent. Today I am thankful to say that several OA members have chosen to move here year-round. We now have a core group to continue the meetings.

I am grateful to my HP and to OA for my recovery and for helping me learn to live life on life's terms without excess food. My life truly is happy, joyous, and free.

❧

It is a higher-powered wonder that I—a single American woman who once lived in fear, fiercely resisted change, took no risks, and hid behind 100 pounds (45 kg) of fat—had the courage to retire to a foreign country where I do not speak the language. I am in awe of my daily good fortune to wake up abstinent in beautiful, semitropical surroundings.

My journey to Mexico began in Overeaters Anonymous meetings in New Jersey twenty-five years ago. There I found a new way of living, and eventually a new life in a new land. All because I was willing to follow a few Steps and suggestions and to give up massive amounts of junk food, which I mistakenly thought I could not live without.

By chance, acquaintances invited me to spend two months avoiding winter weather in a Mexican fishing village. I couldn't pronounce the name of my destination, but I did find it listed on www.oa.org with not one, but two English-speaking meetings. Before my trip, I called the OA contact person who assured me that the basics of my abstinent food plan were available. She agreed to be my temporary sponsor. Today she is my permanent sponsor and a dear friend.

I was nervous about venturing to a strange land with people I barely knew. I almost backed out, but trust in my Higher Power brought me to this place where I know I belong. I returned solo the next winter and was reluctant to leave. Three years ago I obeyed my HP's nudges and made this mountain region my full-time home. Yes, there are challenges and inconveniences. With abstinence and a loving God to guide me, they are manageable and help me accept cultural differences over which I have no control.

The strong OA meetings here were a deciding factor in my move. I need the love, support, and friendship of a recovering community. My new OA family is my lifeline inside and outside the rooms. We are each other's first responders when difficulties strike. There is a group commitment here I have never before experienced. Together we get better—no matter where we compulsive overeaters gather.

❧

I came to OA twenty-four years ago in California and got abstinent within a few months. After five years, I took on more than I could handle. I had a second child and went back to school for a second degree. When I could no longer balance my life, I returned to food, making it my HP. I struggled for many years in and out of relapse. In that time I moved, worked, raised two kids, pursued my second career, and took care of my aging parents. I never stopped going to meetings, although I struggled with surrender and defiance.

Upon retirement, my husband suggested moving to Mexico. I threw up many roadblocks, number one being, "I need my meetings." My husband went to the OA website and found two English-speaking meetings in this location. I figured HP was opening a door for me.

I am so grateful for the people in our small OA group. They have seen me through a series of terrible events: deaths of beloved friends, personal and family illness, the self-inflicted death of a workman in my home while I was in the US and struggles with abstinence. I have really learned that "we will love you until you love yourself." I have seen others go through dark times and remain abstinent. They are my inspiration.

I am coming up on one year here. It has not been easy. I realize that my abstinence is not only important to me, but also to my loving support network in our special little town in Mexico.

I am from Michigan and have been an OA member since 1986. I knew that retirees went to Mexico, but I didn't have an opportunity to do so until after my husband died. I met a widower in 2000, and we decided to check out the expat community I had heard about. I was surprised to find the meetings there in 2001, although they were very small, with only three or four members. I am a snowbird, in Mexico for about seven months a year. When I am back in Michigan, I don't have available face-to-face meetings, so I attend phone meetings!

I think that none of us would recognize each other if the members of my South of the Border groups could meet up with the people we were before we started working the OA program.

I am a recovering anorexic with twenty-four years of abstinence. I moved to Guadalajara, Mexico, from California, knowing there weren't any OA meetings there. Since I wanted to live in Mexico so much, I knew I could start one. I teach Spanish, so I started a Spanish-speaking meeting on Tuesday nights in Guadalajara. I handed out flyers on street corners and put announcements in the newspaper. At one time there were five of us, but the meeting didn't last.

I had registered the meeting with the World Service Office, with me as the contact. One day I got a call from Stephanie, who lived in Ajijic. She wanted to know if there were more meetings in Guadalajara. I told her our meeting had closed, and that I needed a meeting. She told me there were two meetings in her little village. I drove for an hour, met her at a gas station, and followed her to the meeting, which is English-speaking. I've been going now for four years.

I started another meeting in Guadalajara. Sustained by three core members, it lasted almost two years. Then I became pregnant for the first time, with a high-risk pregnancy, needing bed rest. Our second member, whose office hosted our meeting, had to move away. Then came the untimely death of our third member, my beloved fellow OA member and friend, Lety.

Following the premature birth of my daughter, I developed severe, suicidal postpartum depression. I thought I was going to die, despite my love for my husband and new daughter. My OA friends from Ajijic drove back and forth every day to help me remain alive and abstinent. When even this help was not enough, one of them vacated her home in Ajijic so my family and I could move into it. My OA family took turns staying with us practically all day and night. This OA meeting saved my life.

Being befriended by these older OA members has been wonderful for me because I benefit from their experience, strength, and hope on so many things I am going through. Today I am okay. Our daughter has her mom again, and my husband has his wife back. I still drive an hour once, sometimes twice, a week to go to the Ajijic meetings, because without them, I know I would be dead. I love our little group. Thanks to everyone for being willing to be there for me always.

I was shocked to receive the news that my best friend (and first sponsor) had decided to move to Mexico, to some unpronounceable town 3,000 miles (4,828 km) from our home state of New Jersey. This seemed as remote to me as an outpost on the moon. I was almost disbelieving when she told me that her village had two OA meetings a week. We drove together to this unimaginable place for her final move, so I could envision the surroundings in which I was sure she would perish.

She took me to my first Mexican OA meetings. They were held outside in a garden, under a tarp shading us from the sun. We had a lot of "crosstalk" at the meetings: roosters crowing, dogs barking, Spanish music blaring from passing car radios, the clip-clop of horses' hooves on cobblestone streets, as well as trucks with loudspeakers roving the neighborhood announcing their wares in *Español*—produce, water, propane. Periodic explosions from *cohetes* (firework-type rockets) occurred during the many national and religious Mexican fiestas. We also had frequent visits from chickens, hummingbirds, and curious children. Several members brought their dogs, who occasionally added canine comments. When the weather was cool, members would wear colorful rebozos (shawls), emblazoned with the handiwork of the indigenous peoples. When warm, several members would pull out individual straw fans, woven with fabulous colors.

Despite the surreal surroundings, the meetings were the same as they are in the United States. Although small in number (three to twelve members), there were at times six sponsors, many with longtime abstinence. I was humbled to find that my twenty-two years of back-to-back abstinence, maintaining a 100-pound (45-kg) weight loss, was nowhere near others, who had up to thirty years of back-to-back abstinence. Although I was one of only a few who followed a sugar-free, flour-free, volume-free food plan, I was completely at home.

No one was more surprised than I when I rented an apartment

three weeks after my arrival, moving to Mexico at the age of 55, with a disability. I continued to call my sponsor in the US every day to commit my food. I also received a daily call from a sponsee in New Jersey. (My daily gratitude list frequently includes free phone service via the computer.)

The Twelve Traditions are strongly respected, and our groups focus on service and public outreach. A Mexican national, barely speaking English, found recovery in our group. When she established a Spanish-speaking meeting in a nearby village, we donated OA literature translated into Spanish. We supported the establishment of a meeting in Guadalajara, carpooling an hour each way to attend en masse. We now consider ourselves one big group, despite the distance.

We send monthly contributions to the World Service Office and Region Two. We also hope to send a representative to a region conference or the World Service Business Conference in the United States.

To grow our meetings, we place ads in the local English language newspapers and magazines. We post flyers on public bulletin boards and in gyms and leave literature with our physicians. We are registered with the WSO, so we receive calls from OA members visiting or moving to Mexico. We remain connected to our intergroups of origin in Canada and the US, which send newsletters and information.

We share a clubhouse with other Twelve Step fellowships where we hold our meetings. At first, there was no evidence of OA's existence. Today we have an OA literature rack with free pamphlets and a bulletin board displaying the fantastic posters produced by the WSO, plus we distribute free copies of *Lifeline*. Soon to come is an OA sign for the building entrance.

Members of other fellowships comment on the strength of OA recovery, especially our daily use of the Tools. A popular, mixed-fellowship, Twelve Step retreat makes special accommodations for us OA members and our particular food needs. They know that we need access to a kitchen, fridge, and microwave.

We don't consider ourselves survivors in a lifeboat. Instead, we are a family on a pleasure cruise, sailing across our beloved Lake Chapala. Each day we find our sails filled with the loving force of our Higher Power, who is propelling us to our safe harbor of recovery. We welcome all OA travelers seeking the same destination to join us.

We submit this story in loving memory of Lety.

23

Freedom Isn't Free

This year marks thirty years since my first OA meeting. I came and have never left. The miracle happened; today I'm living life, rather than simply enduring it, and holding on to the miracle with a daily routine of actions.

I remember that first meeting well: ten women and me. I had no clue what was going on. I was drunk on food and didn't know it. They were telling stories about their eating and laughing about it, and I didn't quite get what was so funny.

Thirty days earlier, I had written the note, cleaned up my stuff, and in the middle of the night quietly left my home and drove to the bridge. I parked at one end, left my wallet and keys in the car, walked to the center of the bridge, and climbed up on the railing. I stood there, holding onto a wire, needing to take one small step into oblivion.

It was the culmination of obsessing for years about ending my life. I chose the bridge as the most humane way for the sake of my spouse and kids. I would be washed out to sea and become fish food.

I don't know how long I stood there; I don't remember coming down. But I did. Exactly thirty days later I found myself in a room with those ten women. That January night in 1982 was the beginning of a new day, although I was clueless. How did I get there?

In one form or another, fear dominated my life as a child. The figure that most shaped my childhood was a mother who was the seventh child of an alcoholic and raised in poverty in the backwoods of Appalachia. Fear drove her to flee in her early teens to another town, never to return to home or school. With hindsight, I can see that my mother passed her overwhelming fears and insecurities on to me in my childhood. The good news is that fear is learned; therefore, it can be unlearned.

The Christian fundamentalism of my childhood did not serve me well. I was already convinced at age 7 or 8 that I was doomed to hell because I thought bad things, and thinking was as bad as doing. My antagonism toward organized religion festered and grew until I finally began calling myself an atheist.

At age 41, when I came to the program, I was inwardly still the same frightened child, except more so. A lot of years of pretense, role-playing, stroke-seeking, and fear had passed. The result was self-hatred, a feeling of uselessness, and feeling adrift, trapped, and like a victim. All this I felt on the inside despite being a high-functioning, educated person on the outside. This disparity continued for my first forty years until I began to bring the two together through the transformation of the Twelve Steps.

I was not a grossly obese child, though I was always overweight. In high school I played sports and burned up the excess calories I consumed. My compulsive eating began in earnest when I was nineteen and life turned hard. Love broke my heart, and I shut down emotionally for years. I dropped out of college in a drunken stupor, joined the military to escape, quickly met someone, and got married. From the standpoint of maturity, I was stuck somewhere in my mid-teens.

I began to use food as a comfort, escape, and drug. It progressed. It took more and more to get the effect. Two or three donuts became a dozen. A few cookies became the whole package. Half a pizza became a whole pizza. Gradually, eating became almost continuous. I would eat on the way to work, while at work, on the way home from work, then have dinner, sit down in front of the TV, and eat until midnight.

At some point I crossed an invisible line, perhaps in my early 30s. I graduated from simple emotional eater to addict. The genetic predisposition was there, and I had nurtured it to fruition with my excesses. The more I ate, the more I wanted to eat. The first bite set up the urge for more and more. Sugar and refined carbs became for me what alcohol is to an alcoholic. I was addicted, body and soul.

My 20s and 30s were a series of stair-step diets: down and up, down and up, with the up always being more weight. Ultimately my disease took me close to 400 pounds (181 kg), along with the health problems of obesity. After a couple years in OA I was down nearly 200 pounds (91 kg) from my top weight. I regained a few pounds and have now maintained a 185-pound (84-kg) loss for twenty-eight years. My abstinence is three meals a day, nothing in between, no sugar or refined carbs. I weigh and measure when eating at home.

I found my way into OA because I didn't quite have the courage to kill myself. I was grossly obese, suicidal, and of course a bitter atheist. *Other than that, I was fine.*

I argued and argued in those first meetings but really had no place to go. So I finally surrendered to the suggestions. Surrender for me wasn't giving up. It was deciding to cooperate with a new set of ideas about my eating, thinking, and believing. I got abstinent by being willing to admit myself to the metaphorical OA hospital and say, "Okay, I give up. Tell me what to do."

The other OA members told me the first thing to do was to detox from the addictive junk food I was endlessly consuming. I didn't believe in addiction, but I decided to pretend and see what happened. That meant three weighed-and-measured meals a day, no sugar or refined carbohydrates. I figured I couldn't do it all my life, but I would play their game, and when I got thin, I would leave and be able to control it myself.

They told me I was now in a race. What race? It was the race between the eventual decline of my willpower and the acquisition of a new power that would come from working the Twelve Steps. Willpower and the role models in the rooms helped me follow my food plan initially, but other OA members said willpower would eventually run out and had to be replaced by another kind of power. I didn't know what they were talking about, but my pain gave me the willingness to follow directions.

I trusted the process even though I didn't understand it. Eventually I did begin to understand. I had to change how I ate, how I thought, and how I believed. Physically, I had to learn the nature of my food addiction and a new way of eating that keeps it in check. Emotionally, I had to uncover the attitudes, beliefs, and values that are counterproductive to a good life. Spiritually, the Steps took me on a journey to get in touch with the spirit within, which some people call God.

Taking these actions eventually lifted the obsession, as promised in the Big Book. I trusted the process, and the journey took me to spiritual places I could not fathom when I started. Although I call my Higher Power God, part of that HP is still the collective power of the program: the Steps, Traditions, Tools, slogans, and people of the Fellowship. God will guide and give me strength, but he won't do for me what I need to do for myself. God is the well, but I have to bring the bucket of willingness and action.

Holding on to the miracle means staying in fit spiritual condition. It particularly means living in Steps Ten, Eleven, and Twelve. Step Ten is like weeding the garden. I might have done a good job the first time through the Steps, but weeds have a way of creeping back in among the flowers if I don't tend to them continually. The Eleventh Step in the morning is the daily renewal of my faith. If I don't renew my subscription every morning, it runs out sometime during the day. And Step Twelve is about passing it on. To stay clear and clean, a lake needs a flow in and a flow out. My flow-in is working my program. My flow-out is passing on the message to those who are still suffering and practicing these Principles in all my affairs.

Here's one final word on why I'm still here after thirty years—

service. Irish statesman Edmund Burke said, "The only thing necessary for the triumph of evil is for good men to do nothing." I translate that into: The only way for OA to fade away is for people whose lives it has saved to do nothing.

24

PLENTY OF GROWING ROOM LEFT

E ven as a child, I was constantly active and often forgot to eat. By the time I hit puberty, or rather it hit me, fatty padding developed around my breasts and hips. I panicked and attempted to control my weight by obsessively counting calories, weighing myself several times a day, and restricting my food intake to less than nine hundred calories daily. I ruminated constantly about how many calories I had eaten, how long I had gone without eating, when the next meal was coming, and how fat I looked.

In college I suddenly began eating uncontrollably. I had never experienced anything like that. It terrified me. I panicked if I could not get certain foods immediately. I gained over 35 pounds (16 kg), to around 155 pounds (70 kg). At 5 feet 6 and a half inches tall (168 cm), most people thought I looked healthy. But I felt like a worthless, lonely, desperate cow.

I discovered that alcohol diminished my food cravings, but that is another recovery story. I also stumbled into a summer job and realized that heavy, manual labor helped me manage calories without gaining weight. I was hooked. Again, I restricted my food and maintained my weight at a comfortable level.

I thrived on frequent comments such as, "You're so thin!" "I wish I could be that thin," and "I bet you can eat anything you want without gaining weight." My weight constantly yo-yoed 5 or more pounds (2 kg) as I adjusted my food and exercise, repeatedly attempting to eat whatever I wanted without gaining weight. If I gained, I restricted my food until my clothes hung loosely on my body the way I liked them. I constantly worried that I would somehow wake up fat.

In my late 20s, a friend told me about OA. I went to my first meeting in early 1987. I cried through the whole thing. I was blown away that I might have an eating disorder. Though I sat in a room full of overweight men and women, I felt perfectly at home as I listened to them speak of their struggles with food.

Right away, I found a sponsor and began working the Steps. I learned how to eat normally for the first time in my life. God-connection and a huge step of faith helped me begin eating three meals per day, nothing in between, and no sugar. I gained weight without panic. A miracle! I began to heal from a lifetime of vicious self-hatred.

However, my sponsor moved away after a few months. I did not trust people, so I remained shallow with my new sponsor. I stopped sharing my heart and soul in meetings. I resorted to "talking the talk." I sat in meetings another four years spouting what I thought *others* needed to hear, cleverly cloaked in my own "I statements." I ached with loneliness but could not ask for help. After a while I doubted my need for OA since I was getting so little out of it, and I made a conscious decision to leave for a shallow life.

In 1992 I moved to a new town and stopped going to meetings. Effortlessly, I justified eating white flour and sugar again. I also discovered a new drug: bicycling. Soon, I was riding my bicycle up to fourteen hours per week, up to nine hours a ride.

In January 1994, I finally faced that I could not manage refined sugar. I weaned myself off of it, and by God's grace I have not had it since. However, in order to cycle all those hours, I had to consume a lot of food. Although I avoided refined sugar, my eating was far from sane. My life revolved around exercise, food, and body image.

In 2000 a miracle happened. I developed health challenges, and one night in August, I tallied the ample evidence that exercise had become my god. I thought of all the times I failed to cut back on exercise, all the things I let go for exercise, how I evaluated everything around how much exercise I could incorporate, and how I required exorbitant amounts of food in order to exercise at that level. Finally, by God's grace, I admitted the truth. I knew OA was the solution.

I came back into the rooms desperate enough to do whatever it took to recover. I found a wonderful sponsor, who is still my sponsor, and began working the Steps, calling her regularly, baring my soul to her and in meetings, and attending several meetings per week. After all these years, I still read OA literature daily, journal, develop a daily gratitude list, make regular program calls, attend several meetings per week, sponsor others, and practice and apply the Steps in all my affairs.

One of the most helpful slogans I heard when I came in was, "We're only as sick as the secrets we keep." I pray before every meeting that God will help me say what I need to say, because left to my own devices, I will hide. My medicine is to say aloud the very things my disease tells me to bury.

In recovery, I have experienced many profound healings. Abandonment, abuse, postabortion grief, denial of my lesbian sexuality, paralyzing fear of people, frozen emotions, rigid Christianity, and the illusion that God had abandoned me—these rose to the surface for healing as I embraced the gift of sanity with food and exercise. Compassion and understanding are now replacing the raging self-hatred that had maimed me. Ever-deepening surrender is slowly replacing my self-will. A faithful, loving God is replacing the rigid distortion I had held as a deity. Trust is replacing fear.

After a life-threatening car accident, I hit my lowest weight of less than 100 pounds (45 kg) since returning to OA. Recovery has been imperfect and slow for me, but I go at my own pace because I know genuine healing takes time. Today, I weigh around 112 pounds (51 kg), a weight that would previously have panicked me. I continue to grow in accepting my body as it is.

My life today revolves around deepening connections with God and others, rather than around exercise, food, or body image. I weigh monthly, refuse calorie counting, and follow a food and exercise plan, as I have for years. These are not my accomplishments, but rather miraculous gifts of God through OA.

I could never have imagined the freedom from food, exercise, and body obsession I know today. I continue to heal on all levels, but I am a million times better than I was before OA. This is the only place I have found the tools I need to live without regressing into the insanity that drove me here in the first place.

I am deeply grateful for this program. I believe it can work for anyone, even me. Since I have plenty of growing room left, I keep coming back.

25

A BLACK COMPULSIVE OVEREATER WHO FOUND HER SOUL

For fifty years, starting at 18 months of age, I ate compulsively and got progressively worse. Before I came to Overeaters Anonymous, I experienced overeating, bulimia, and anorexia. I was a physical wreck. When I got to 230 pounds (104 kg), I refused to weigh myself anymore. I was taking medication for hypertension and my cholesterol was above 300. I was emotionally and mentally challenged and taking psychotropic medication. I was spiritually bankrupt, although I was very religious.

When I came to OA at the age of 53, I was so depressed I wanted to die. Now, I am grateful that my religious beliefs meant suicide was not an option. In OA, I have found a way to actually live according to my beliefs.

My father died when I was 33. I was so disturbed by his death that a doctor committed me to a mental hospital and diagnosed me with bipolar disorder. For the next twenty years I lost and regained a hundred pounds (45 kg) several times. I was in and out of the mental hospital because I played games with the medication.

When I came to OA, I got honest about what I was doing and

became willing to take the medications as prescribed. As a result, my condition stabilized and has remained that way. A reading titled "How It Works" from the Big Book says, "There are those, too, who suffer from grave emotional and mental disorders, but many of them do recover if they have the capacity to be honest" (*Alcoholics Anonymous*, 4th ed., p. 58). This materialized in my life and is truly a miracle.

Desperation led me to my first contact with OA. I believe I arrived already "surrendered." So, without knowing, I was abstinent when I got to my first meeting. I had found the missing piece of the puzzle, and I was home. I got a sponsor and started working the Steps. I have written more than seven Fourth Steps over the fourteen years I have been in the program. During the first two years I was also in psychotherapy. I had been in and out of therapy for twenty years without much success, but therapy and working the program worked for me. I still see my therapist once a month for maintenance and my psychiatrist monitors my medication.

For the first three years my weight loss was amazing. As I worked the Steps the weight just seemed to fall off. Then I experienced a life crisis that ended my thirty-eight year marriage. The emotional pain was so great that I became willing to accept a food plan. I began to weigh and measure my food, and for the first time, I realized that how much I weigh relates to how much I eat. Before that I did not have a clue.

After five and a half years in the program, I broke my abstinence at a holiday party where I ate the desserts. So I started over. It took me ten years to lose a 100 pounds (45 kg), which was a blessing in disguise because it gave me time to change my eating habits.

Soul food was the comfort food that I returned to after I finished any diet. But this time was different. When I got to goal weight in the program, I started following a food plan for maintenance. With the help of my maintenance sponsor, I have been at goal weight for three and a half years. Continually working the Twelve Steps, abiding by the Twelve Traditions, and giving service at meetings are integral to that maintenance.

OA has both saved me and given me a life. Before OA the food kept me numb; I felt neither the pain nor the joy of life. I no longer seek comfort or escape through food. Now, food sustains me and allows me to live more actively. I am open to all the joys, pains, and subtleties of life. Last year, when my mother passed, abstinence and the Twelve Steps allowed me to feel the loss without turning to comfort foods and without hospitalization or more medicine.

I have been retired for more than a year. My life is now about doing service both in and out of OA. I continue to provide clinical supervision for young people working toward licensure in the profession from which I retired. It is a way to give back to my profession and to others. I do service and sponsor both in OA and another Twelve Step program. I especially enjoy sponsoring newcomers. These are ways to bring life to an old adage, "Freely ye have received, so freely give."

If I had not come to OA when I did, I do not believe I would have lived to get old enough to retire. I have financial challenges from time to time, but I now have a life that is beyond my wildest dreams.

26

TWELVE KEYS

L ooks like you've let yourself go over the summer," my college friend said. I shrugged my shoulders and left for class. I was mortified, for I had not casually put on 34 pounds (15 kg). I had worked at it.

Scads of empty candy wrappers revealed my bingeing. I had searched for the excitement of the first compulsive bite, long after it was past. Sugar gave me release from care and relief from craving. I felt like a heroin addict must feel. I would think, "I've eaten so much, I'll just finish the box." Never mind that I couldn't cross my legs or that my boyfriend called me "Thunder Thighs." The reasons for the binges were less important than the consequences. If I had an ounce of self-pity at the start of that summer, I had tons of self-hate at the end.

It took me four years to lose what I had gained in only three months. After I graduated, a peer exclaimed, "You've lost weight!" I replied, "Yes, but it's just a matter of time before I gain it back." He said, "I've been going to Overeaters Anonymous. You should try it."

I denied that my behavior was a symptom of a physical, emotional, and spiritual disease, but I did admit I wasn't eating normally. As *The Twelve Steps and Twelve Traditions of Overeaters Anonymous* says on page 2, "Like compulsive overeaters, normal eaters will sometimes find pleasure and escape from life's problems in excess food. Compulsive overeaters, however, often have an abnormal reaction when we overindulge. We can't quit. A normal eater gets full and loses interest in food. We compulsive overeaters crave more." Having family members see me sneaking ice cream or having sugar on my shirt at an OA meeting was embarrassing. Still, shame did not help me abstain. Once I dieted to extreme. A photo shows me sitting on a dock with my pale, bony shoulders hunched forward. I look weak and wasted.

After thirteen years of working as a nurse, an injury disabled me. I could not sit, stand, or walk for longer than ten minutes, and for ten years I stuffed the anger down with food. Finally, I was desperate enough to call an OA member named Kay and ask her to be my sponsor. I envied her for her small size and straight talk. At the time, she had been abstinent for fifteen years. The fact that she used the OA Tools, worked the Twelve Steps and Twelve Traditions, had a working knowledge of the Twelve Concepts, and did service was lost on me. All I knew was that she was my last chance.

I was trying to cope with job loss, child rearing, and the family disease of alcoholism, so I thought I had plenty to do. But Kay wanted me to write down a food plan and my feelings every day, and to call her periodically. "When will I have time?" I asked. "You'll make time," she said.

One day Kay asked me, "What do all addicts fear the most?" I couldn't guess. "Change," she replied. "In OA, you put down the fork and pick up the Steps. You work all twelve in order and you will never have to overeat again—if you don't want to."

I feared failure, but I got abstinent within two years of working with her. I thoroughly took the first Step, admitting I was powerless over food and my life had become unmanageable. But I balked when I was working on the Second and Third Steps, as described in OA's *Twelve and Twelve*, "Some of us walked out of our first meeting when we heard that three-letter word mentioned." (*The Twelve Steps and Twelve Traditions of Overeaters Anonymous,* p. 13). I initially felt that God was concerned only with morality and eternal life, but I finally came to believe there was a power greater than myself who could restore me to sanity. I might as well call this power God. Kay suggested that my God was not very caring, and offered me hers.

Every time I wanted to take a break from the Twelve Steps, Kay would be patient or prompt me forward. I didn't want to bare my soul, but after writing my Fourth Step inventory, I read it to her. She kindly accepted me and did not make me feel guilty. She lovingly confronted me with the character defects that kept me stuck. While she encouraged that I take on the humility of Step Seven, she told me to take off my "Mother Teresa cap" when I got fixated on perfection.

When I hung on to self-pity, she said my new nursing position was to play "special teams" when needed. Indeed, I have called 911 twice for family members. Making the direct amends of Step Nine was worth the solace it gave me. Now I am glad to admit mistakes rather than let animosity or guilt build. Each afternoon I set aside time for the prayer and meditation of Step Eleven, so I can connect with this God I now love.

This year I will have twelve years of abstinence. I almost never have a craving for extra food. I am at a normal weight for my height. As wonderful as it was to throw away my green "fat pants," the best thing is my growing ability to live life on life's terms. This has not always been easy.

Last year, my 58-year-old husband had a stroke. He had a headache on Friday and died on Sunday. Before I left the hospital Saturday night, I kissed him goodbye and said, "I'll see you in the morning," and he replied, "Okay." Those were our last words. I did not overeat or starve then or now. How? I didn't do it alone. I accepted the hugs of my sponsor and other OA friends. I also pictured myself crawling into the loving lap of my Higher Power, whom I call God. I could not have been strong for my children if I had not been abstinent. Kay reminds me, "Some days are just trudge days." My life is not a "happy ever after," but there is happiness in each day, and the good days keep coming.

I love being abstinent. The Steps require willingness, persistence, and continuous action, but that is a small price to pay for joy. Phone calls, sponsorship, food plans, literature, anonymity, action plans, meetings, writing, and service have enabled me to leave my prison of shame behind.

I sponsor now, and I try to pass on the twelve keys of freedom—one for every Step—to others. If you are a newcomer, keep coming back. If you are a struggling longtimer, keep coming back. We have a set of keys with your name on it.

27

SURRENDER BRINGS FREEDOM

For as long as I can remember, my mind has been obsessed with eating, dieting, and exercising. Round and round my thoughts would go, questioning everything that had to do with food and how to get thin. Which meal choice had the least amount of calories? How much would I have to exercise to stay thin if I ate three candy bars? I'm already fat and alone; what does it matter if I eat the whole pizza and have ice cream for dessert?

Counting calories, using laxatives to lose weight, starving myself and then bingeing until I felt like I was going to vomit—it was exhausting. By the time I found OA, I was 5 feet 4 inches (162 cm) and over 260 pounds (118 kg). I had tried everything else to control my eating and weight, only to discover that none of it worked. No diet, therapist, exercise, or drug was ever able to keep me from diving into a bag of cookies and finishing the whole thing.

When I was a teenager, I even prayed to become anorexic or bulimic. I saw TV movies about those girls and the places they could go to find help. I tried again and again to make myself throw up, but for whatever reason, my gag reflexes wouldn't allow me to do it. And starving myself was never an option. I couldn't stop eating, no matter how hard I tried. I was tired of trying and failing. I was depressed, angry, alone, morbidly obese, and hopeless.

I attended my first OA meeting in August 1999 at the suggestion of a counselor. I was 29 years old. I sat in a room with mostly thin women, wondering what they were doing there.

When the meeting started and they began sharing their stories, I couldn't believe what I heard. Everything they said about what they had done with food or how their minds obsessed on food was something I had done or thought. For the longest time, I had believed I was the only person who did these things with food. I thought other fat people had health problems or slow metabolisms, and I was just weak willed. Hearing other people talk about the things I had done with food and dieting jolted me into a state of hope. Could it be true? Was there actually a solution for someone like me? Absolutely!

For me OA was—and is—the only solution to my food obsession. When I tried to argue with my sponsor about my food plan, she asked me, "Jessica, are you willing to try something different?" That question stopped me dead in my tracks. All my arguments seemed to slip away. God granted me surrender and willingness. The suggestions of my sponsor and other abstinent OA members became my Higher Power without me even knowing it.

They told me to write down my food plan and call someone for help if anything changed. Making decisions about food on my own had only ever gotten me fat and unhappy; why not try something different? They told me to go to meetings and get involved in service to help enhance the Fellowship of OA. Sitting at home by myself watching TV had only ever gotten me fat and unhappy; why not try something different? They told me to reach out to other members and ask for help in living the Twelve Step program one day at a time. Trying to figure things out on my own had only ever gotten me fat and unhappy; why not try something different?

So, I tried something different—and it worked! In the first two years of my abstinence, I lost 120 pounds (54 kg) and have kept it off ever since. Not only has the program given me a healthy physical body, but it has also given me emotional sobriety and a spiritual connection that is beyond my wildest dreams. I am no longer tired, depressed, angry, alone, or hopeless. Through working the Steps with my sponsor and applying the Principles of those Steps in my daily life, my obsession with food has been lifted and I have learned how to accept life as it is, one day at a time.

I wish I could say that every moment in OA has been all peaches and cream (pun intended), but it hasn't. As wonderful as God's grace has been in granting me surrender and willingness, this Twelve Step program of recovery is not always easy. My ego, pride, and self-righteousness are constantly trying to find their way back into my daily life. They sit, watch, and wait for an opportunity when my defenses are down and then they strike.

Maybe I've stopped going to meetings regularly or I'm dragging my feet on a writing assignment from my sponsor. Maybe I've stopped doing service because I'm "too busy." Maybe I've forgotten to pray for a few days in a row. That's when the door opens, and those character defects enter with gusto. Sometimes they come out sideways when I speak harshly to a family member.

Other times they come out front and center by renewing my cravings for my binge foods. Either way, they put me in the danger zone. At that point, I either turn back to the program or I face relapse. When I face this choice, I am forever grateful to other OA members who have shared their honest experience, strength, and hope at OA meetings. Those who have experienced relapse and come back willing to share the pain of breaking their abstinence and the difficulty in getting it back have given me a priceless asset in keeping my abstinence intact. And those members who have stayed abstinent and remind me that relapse is not a requirement for OA membership have also given me a hope I never knew was possible.

The difficult moments when my disease fights back have helped me recognize there is no graduation day from working the Twelve Steps and using the OA Tools. I believe I will never see the day when I can walk away from OA and stay clean. I also believe that in order to keep my abstinence and continue to grow emotionally and spiritually, I must continue to be honest with myself and my sponsor, commit my food regularly, ask for help, offer help to others, and have a plan.

As I continue to surrender to the Twelve Steps and the Tools of this program, I continue to be free. It is that simple.

28

CONQUERING THE ABCS

By the grace of my Higher Power, I am recovering from this deadly disease. I have the ABCs of eating disorders—Anorexia: I used to starve myself, sometimes for days in a row; Bulimia: I used to purge the excess weight through laxative abuse and overexercising; and Compulsive overeating: before I came to OA in 2001 at the age of 42, I ate myself up to at least 437 pounds (198 kg), wearing pants with a 66-inch (168-cm) waist.

I had lost the weight many times before I came to OA, but the Twelve Steps are the only thing that has allowed the weight to stay off. I am now 52 years old, 5 feet 10 inches (177 cm) tall, wear pants with a 36-inch (91-cm) waist, and have weighed in the 160-pound (73-kg) range for the last nine years. My current abstinence date is July 28, 2002. God-given abstinence is the most important thing in my life without exception.

I am happy most of the time, and I choose to send that message to my face more often. I have received so much from OA, and that reminds me to give back to OA with service.

So what was I like? I was filled with self-hatred and didn't want anyone to know. Most of my life I allowed others to influence me, and I was constantly seeking approval. I never felt I was good enough. (BINGE is a good acronym for Because I'm Not Good Enough.)

My concept of God was punitive. Most of the time I experienced the driving need to overeat. When I graduated from grade school, my mother had the baker write on the cake, "To the Superior, Inferior Child" (not "Congratulations!"). I asked her why. She said, "Well, you think you're so superior, but you're really inferior." She was right. I did feel (and act) that way, but I thought I was fooling people. I remember going out with friends in 1982 and stealing food off the table to take with me for "later." At that point one friend said, "Please don't; we think so highly of you." Who, me? Why would anyone think highly of me? I felt worthless.

I tried many ways to control my weight: crazy diets, commercial food plans, exercising (sometimes even with a vinyl sweatsuit on; remember those dangerous things?). Most of these involved the use of willpower. Using willpower is about as effective for the disease of compulsive overeating as it is for cancer. I basically had two main thoughts: Food was the main one, and the other was IWIWD, my code for I Wish I Were Dead.

What happened? In 1998, a friend sent me a book about Overeaters Anonymous and shared that she had gone to OA meetings but had not stuck with it. She thought all the Steps were great, except Step One; she refused to abstain from a certain food that she just had to have. Back then, I wanted no part of OA.

The next year, in 1999, my 14-year-old son passed away suddenly, and the doctors never figured out why. Oh sure, they put something on the death certificate but couldn't find it on the autopsy. I overate over that. It didn't help. Then I dieted myself down to about 180 pounds (82 kg).

In 2001, after planes flew into buildings in New York City and elsewhere, I decided to go to my first OA meeting on Thanksgiving Day (two months after the planes and over three years after my friend first carried the message to me). I heard people share, and I was immediately convinced I had this disease, but these people could never understand me. I talked to no one, bought forty dollars worth of literature, and left, telling myself I would not return.

I came back to another special OA event (as the Thanksgiving marathon of meetings was) on what I now know to be Unity Day. I listened to the speakers; one of them asked for my phone number, and without thinking, I gave it to her. A while later, she called me. I couldn't believe it! I still remember that person and that call. Of course, I called no one. I started going infrequently to a local meeting and was abstinent off and on for about eight months. When I did show up, I cried (I didn't even care that I was a guy crying in front of a bunch of women).

I knew I was in pain—severe pain. That was my motivator. The first seven months of 2002, I attended my home meeting three times. I started abstinence many times. There were days when I ate about 14,000 calories worth of food (my best guess). At one point, I gained 40 pounds (18 kg) in three weeks, going from about 180 pounds (82 kg) to 220 pounds (100 kg). Then I starved myself, trying to be "good." I just couldn't work this program (on my own that is). Then, on July 28, 2002, I accepted the gift of abstinence again and said to myself, "This will never work, but there's one way to find out—by doing it."

What am I like now? Abstinence (a gift from my Higher Power) is the most important thing in my life without exception. Without it, I don't believe I would have a life worth living. I am abstaining from the foods and behaviors that cause me problems. I follow a food plan that includes a variety of foods that taste good to me. I choose to weigh and measure most of my food in some way. How do I know if any nutritionally sound food plan is working? If I am eating to approach or maintain a healthy body weight, then it's working.

Certain foods are better off in the trash than on my body. A food plan by itself, however, is not enough. I need the spirituality that OA offers. I need God and the help only other OA members can give.

Other than the foods and behaviors that cause me problems, here's a list of some other things I get to abstain from as well: shortness of breath while sitting still; mental fog; food hangovers; having breasts larger than some women; stinking from poor hygiene habits; eating spoiled food; the feeling of being poisoned, ill, and sweaty most of the time; breaking chairs; sneaking food; the frightening humiliation of being out of control; a sticky steering wheel in my car; frequent food stains on seat belts and clothes.

I try to cooperate with my Higher Power now. I accept that compulsive overeating is not an option. I am simply your brother on the journey we are all on. I ignore the craving; it rarely comes. I work on my posture and attitude. I practice self-care by making my bed, combing my hair, brushing and flossing my teeth. I pray, thanking God for all that I've been given. I make calls to my sponsor and others. I try to live the Steps, not just work them. I go to meetings.

I don't remember all the meetings I've attended or readings I've enjoyed, just as I don't remember every single abstinent meal I've ever had. But I am sure they've all nourished me. I want to live a fulfilling life, so for right now, I am choosing to move in that direction. Only then can I be of service to God and other people. It's much better to enlarge my spiritual life than my physical body once again.

29

AGONY AUNT SAVED MY LIFE

In 1985 I was diagnosed with amenorrhea, the absence of a menstrual period in a woman of reproductive age. I faced hospitalization if my weight fell any lower. I was 5.5 stone (35 kg; 77 lbs).

How did it all begin? As a child I could eat anything and not put on weight. I was of Jamaican origin, and I was a loner who kept to myself. My nickname at home was "Bones" and at school "The Biafran."

At 18 my prayers were answered, and I went to university in the north of England. Away from London and my parents' strict home, I had my first taste of excess. I studied engineering and was one of five girls in a class of forty men. As a young, thin black woman considered pretty by many, I worked to extremes and partied hard. But I had few friends and was the subject of many men's interests, and terrible racism at the university. I consoled myself in the lap of excess drinking, food, and relationships.

On leaving university, I worked at an international oil company, but I struggled to make an impression on my manager. I lived alone and eventually stopped eating properly because of work pressures. I would "suck" on healthy food: chew, inhale, and not swallow certain foods. People started to draw attention to my weight, and I liked it. If I could sculpt my body through starvation and look pretty, maybe people would appreciate me.

I resigned from the job and moved back in with my father to care for him as he underwent an operation. During this period, I suffered the sudden death of near relatives. I underate and compulsively exercised to cope with the intense pain of loss. I discovered that I could vomit with ease, and I was disgusted with myself after each episode. If I was unhappy with regurgitation, I would take up to thirty laxatives per day.

Eventually my periods stopped. I was referred to a consultant at a leading hospital, who offered psychotherapy and threatened me with hospitalization. I had successfully secured a new job and the fear of not working galvanized me to eat excessively. My anorexia morphed into bulimia.

I thought I was evil and went to a priest for a prayer to remove the evil within me. The priest gently told me I was not evil, but very unwell and should see a doctor.

During psychotherapy, the young, handsome psychotherapist would sometimes finish a packet of food in front of me while I did all the speaking. I watched him consume food, enjoyed his handsome, Hollywood-actor face, and after the session, I ate whole bags of sugar-laden, full-fat food. Then I regurgitated multiple times per evening until sometimes I drew blood.

Twice I realized I was about to pass out when driving because of my low weight, so I had to pull over to the side of the road. Eventually I would eat something and continue driving. I ate frozen food and stale food covered in mold. I would run across a busy road at 1:00 a.m. to buy tubs of ice cream to eat. Each day I would go to work, function, and then go home to hell.

One day, full of remorse and exhausted after multiple bulimic episodes, I got down on my knees and prayed, "God, if there truly is a God, please heal me of this food disorder. I don't know how long I have to live. Please stop me from doing this."

I switched on the radio and heard a well-known agony aunt giving advice on medical problems. I called the program and was placed on air. I revealed everything, and she introduced me to Overeaters Anonymous. After the radio call ended, my father called and asked if that was me on the radio. I replied, Yes. He said, "Come home."

My father, sisters, and mother wept and said they would do everything in their power to help me. It was 1988. I walked into my first grey sheet meeting on a Saturday in London. When I heard the beautiful women sharing their testimony, they shared my story and I wept. When they mentioned a Higher Power, I realized God had answered my prayer and brought me home.

I received a sponsor that day, and she spent time after the meeting purchasing scales and measuring cups for a food plan. I had forgotten what a portion size was and completely surrendered to her food plan. We agreed that I would call in my food each day. I was eternally grateful for the accountability.

In my first year I slipped up several times and had awful binges. I worked the Steps with my sponsor, and she had a great faith. Individuals were celebrated and received recovery coins for their back-to-back abstinence. I hungered for recovery because I was still slipping and sliding. I got down on my knees and prayed hard for abstinence and well-being.

Then one day I became abstinent. After seven years of grey sheet, I found a new sponsor where my food plan evolved to a high carbohydrate, high fruit, and vegetables food plan without weighing and measuring. After several years of sponsoring, being sponsored, and almost ten years of back-to-back abstinence, and performing a variety of service positions, I left OA in 1998.

Three years of hell ensued, and my bulimia was progressive, rampant, and at times, unstoppable. In 2001 I rediscovered OA and never looked back.

In 2007 my mother died of cancer, my mother who had weighed and measured my food in early recovery. I miss her and thank God for my abstinence throughout the pain and loss.

I am maintaining a 2.5-stone (16-kg, 35-lb) weight gain. However, with the help of the medical profession, God, and accountability to my sponsor, I am embracing more changes in my physical, emotional, and spiritual recovery in the form of an action plan. In my 48 years, God has done for me what I could not do for myself. I thank God for the discovery of OA and my life.

30

OUT OF DARKNESS

I believe I was genetically predisposed to addiction; it ran in my family. Growing up, I was fixated on sugar. When my mother was cookie chairman for a youth organization, I stole many boxes of cookies, ate them, and hid the empty boxes under my bed. I was eight years old. By the age of twenty, I had become emotionally dependent on food. I was a single parent on welfare, living in my parents' dysfunctional home. I had dropped out of school when I had my son. Food was my way of dealing with the hurt and shame I felt.

I returned to school at my parents' insistence, but I never felt like I fit in with the other students, and food continued to be my solace. I was up to 165 pounds (75 kg) and unhappy with my appearance. I first went to OA looking for a diet. It was the only one I could afford. I followed a very strict food plan, lost about 25 pounds (11 kg), and left the rooms after a couple of months.

After graduating, I got a job and got off welfare. My security and sense of self-worth came solely from my job. For the first nine years, I burned the candle at both ends, and feeling self-pity for how hard I worked, I rewarded myself with food. The words from *The Twelve Steps and Twelve Traditions of Overeaters Anonymous*, "We worked hard during the day and ate hard at night" (p. 11) described me perfectly.

During this time I had moved out of my parents' house and my eating really came on strong. I now had privacy to go with my paycheck, and I didn't have to worry about hiding junk food in my purse or under my coat when I returned from the store. I battled my weight using commercial diets, but by 1998 I was approaching 200 pounds (91 kg). My life had become unmanageable. I was a neglectful parent. I was constantly paying bills late, which wrecked my credit and resulted in my landlord not renewing my apartment lease. I had to move back in with my parents. I felt like a failure, and again I turned to OA to help with the food, but also to help with my emotions.

I got emotional support from the friends I found in OA. I enjoyed the meetings, and again had physical recovery, losing around 40 pounds (18 kg). But I wasn't using all the Tools or working the Steps, so after a fight with my mother, I impulsively moved out. Shortly afterward, I was back into the food. Over the next five months, I regained all the weight and then some.

A year later, after struggles at work, I felt my job was threatened. By this time, my weight was well over 200 pounds (91 kg), and I was ill prepared for a job search at that size. So in 2000 I returned to OA again, very motivated. I hit meetings, got my first sponsor, committed my food, read literature, did writing, used the telephone, and did service. This time I lost 70 pounds (32 kg). I thought I was working the program, but I wasn't working the Steps. After five months of abstinence, I felt I wanted a break from the hard work of recovery and left OA. I quickly put on 80 pounds (36 kg) and my disease went to a new level.

I was out of the rooms for seven years, and my disease progressed to the point where I ate only in binges. After I passed the 300 pound (136 kg) mark, my brother did a mini-intervention and got me back to an OA meeting. I realized I had to do something different to get a different result; I needed to work the Steps. So I formed a Step study group that met at my house.

Over the next several months, I worked the Steps. I was able to forgive myself and others and made some amends. During this time, I lost 60 pounds (27 kg) and began to heal my relationship with my Higher Power. However, I still just couldn't surrender all to God. After about nine months I relapsed yet again.

I then experienced what I call The Dark Year. I was so deep in the food, I couldn't see out of the pit. I was bingeing nonstop, only to sleep. I had food stashed everywhere. I had no social life. My knees hurt. I had sleep apnea and high blood pressure. I couldn't fit in airplane seats. I had sores that took a long time to heal. I was killing myself, pure and simple. At 311 pounds (141 kg), I stopped weighing myself.

In October 2010, my mentor at work was fired. With him gone, I felt vulnerable. I had slacked off quite a bit over the years. I knew I had to do something, not just about my weight but also about my life. My Higher Power intervened. He gave me strong direction to return to OA, but I was scared I wouldn't be able to put the food down. The food voices were shouting in my head all day. They had to stop for me to have a chance to work the program. In prayer, I begged God to silence the voices in my head. No sooner had I spoken those words than the voices were gone. It was a true miracle. I got abstinent that day, went to a meeting, got a sponsor, and began working the Steps immediately.

Ten days later the food voices returned, and I picked up. I couldn't believe I had picked up so soon. I was very scared. I knew my premature death was waiting for me outside the rooms. I *ran* to God. I was ready to surrender my life. I laid bare my heart and soul to God, holding nothing back. I begged him for help. I was instantly filled with a peace that brought tears to my eyes. I have never been that happy in my life. I was complete. The pit was not filled—it was gone.

God has directed my life since then. It's been full of joy and usefulness. I've celebrated a year of abstinence and transformed from size 32 to size 18. On a daily basis, I work with my sponsor and sponsees, from whom I am learning so much about myself and my Higher Power. I perform service at the intergroup level and am ready to take on service at the region level.

Does this mean every day is easy? No. I still have food thoughts and occasionally get cravings. I know my disease is right there, like a shark cruising under the surface waiting for an opportunity to strike. I must protect myself from getting too hungry, angry, lonely, or tired. I must stay honest. I must make amends for any harm I've caused. I must surrender myself to God every day, throughout the day. I must always remember that, for me, OA is not optional. It is keeping me alive and is filling my life with love and understanding beyond my wildest dreams.

31

THE BEST DEFENSE OF ALL

I'm a 58-year-old male and have been in OA since February 1990. During my first five years in OA, I had incidental but regular slips. When I fully surrendered and became willing to receive everything the program had to offer, my life began to change, and it has continued to change for the better ever since. I've been binge-free since I joined OA in 1990, but my last willful, impulsive, or defiant compulsive bite was on January 30, 1996.

My story is not particularly unique. Early on, I developed a liking for favorite foods and went to increasing lengths to get them. This benign habit of chasing a pleasing taste soon became a ritual of escape from my feelings and responsibilities. My normal emotional development suffered because I demanded more from food than it was ever intended to provide.

I was an emotional and impulsive child. I reacted to life with fear, anxiety, and aggression. I was ashamed of my emotions; they seemed so big. When I ate foods with flour and sugar in them, it seemed to dull my feelings. Much of the time I was under the influence of my last foray into the food, or reeling from the physical and emotional aftermath of having eaten compulsively. I didn't know it at the time. It's just the way things were.

I also suffered from attention deficit disorder and didn't feel like I fit in anywhere. I didn't trust easily, believing that once people got close to me, they would see how weird I was and tell the rest of the world. This was just one of many lies that my mind used to keep me trapped in a defensive posture and a perpetual cycle of relief-seeking.

I was athletic and quite thin in my early life. However, given my insecurities, I used my skills to competitively abuse my opponents, presumably to feel better about myself. I frequently incurred injuries and rushed back before they had properly healed—anything to avoid sitting still. I suffered from chronic aches and pains and slowly realized I was losing the battle of controlling my weight through sports and exercise.

I was preoccupied with the size and shape of my body, yet I was terribly judgmental of heavy people. How ironic that years later, many of the answers to my food problem would come from the very people I had held in contempt for so long.

As I got older, my addictions grew to include drugs, alcohol, and sex. If something felt good, I used it until it didn't work anymore. My chances for healthy, intimate relationships were severely damaged by the selfishness and immaturity that goes hand in hand with addiction.

Eventually, my Higher Power saw fit to send a recovering alcoholic into my life. Through my relationship with her, I found my way into a Twelve Step program in 1983. I'd never seen anything like her devotion to staying sober and her willingness to deal with life a day at a time. She spoke honestly about her past and clearly was anchored to something solid and substantial. That kind of courage gave me hope.

Eventually I sobered up and began working my program, but I struggled with resentment and continued to blame others for my problems because I was still in the food. I was holding back, and I lacked the humility to fully take Step One.

Fifteen months into sobriety, I started dating another woman who eventually entered several Twelve-Step fellowships, including OA. When I became ready, she gently guided me to OA. We recently celebrated our twenty-fifth wedding anniversary.

I never became obese and am maintaining a 30 to 35 pound (14 to 16 kg) weight loss. However, it was clear to me that I didn't have to be fat to be a food addict. My emotional and spiritual emptiness ultimately drove me to my bottom and into OA.

I needed to check my ego at the door, unlearn a lot of what I thought I knew from my other Twelve Step fellowship, and take Step One all over again. "How it Works" from the Big Book says, "If you have decided you want what we have and are willing to go to any length to get it, then you are ready to take certain steps" (*Alcoholics Anonymous*, 4th ed., p. 58). The if/then nature of that proposition eluded me for quite a while as I selectively picked and chose the things I was willing to do.

It took me five years in OA before I gained continuous abstinence. I had to surround myself with OA members who were committed to that goal each and every day; people who treated the first compulsive bite like a sober alcoholic treated the first drink. As long as I believed I could willfully jump back and forth over the blurry line that was my initial abstinence, I would continue to fail. I had to stop fighting the diagnosis and embrace the solution.

Before program, I had no spiritual dimension in my life. I was born Jewish, but that meant nothing to me. Now I am an Orthodox Jew, largely because my abstinence came to depend on learning to integrate structure, take direction, respect the need for clear boundaries, and be honest about whether I was living in personal integrity. These actions and principles prepared me to embrace the stringencies of my religious heritage, all of which bring me closer to God.

The Steps have fulfilled their promise of completely changing my outlook. I see my resistance to working any of the Tools on a given day as the first sign of my next compulsive bite. I am very active in OA service, so I am never far from memories of my early difficulties in trying to gain balance in my life.

I believe my Higher Power gives me everything I need to meet the challenges of the day with courage and acceptance. I now see adversity as an opportunity to grow spiritually, not as punishment for being a loser.

I firmly believe that OA's future success rests squarely on the shoulders of tomorrow's sponsors. Even one generation of weak sponsorship will produce a pale shadow of the best that OA has to offer. If I cannot convey practical ways for a newcomer to stay abstinent on a daily basis and prepare him or her to walk through the Twelve Steps with a sense of optimism, I don't believe I have fulfilled my OA responsibility.

I have been given back the choice to eat compulsively or not, and I fully understand what I stand to lose if I fail to acknowledge this gift each day. By starting each morning being grateful for this beautiful life, I am cultivating the best defense of all against the first compulsive bite.

32

I Came on My Hands and Knees

I am a compulsive overeater and food addict. I'm also a person with a mental illness, and I am a lesbian. I have always been accepted in OA because the gender of the person one falls in love with doesn't matter; compulsive overeating kills us all. By the grace of God, I will soon have three years of abstinence.

I've been a compulsive overeater since I was 5 years old. My mother sent me to kindergarten with a snack and warned me not to eat too much, but I couldn't stop. I went on my first diet at age eight. During my teen years, I ate twelve slices of bread a day. In my 20s, I took karate for six years and ate fiercely. Even though I trained six days a week, I had a belly.

In my early 30s, I had a nervous breakdown and went on disability. When I stopped the karate, I continued to overeat. I ballooned up to over 200 pounds (91 kg). I began taking prescribed medications, and I went up to 310 pounds (141 kg).

I got a job tuning pianos part-time and began going to a day treatment program, which helped. But I still continued to eat too much. I ate when I was happy, angry, sad, and lonely, and when I wanted to celebrate or reward myself. Food was my answer for anything that happened. I did not realize until I became abstinent that I had made food my Higher Power. Only God could remove this kind of thinking, and she did.

I came into the program on my hands and knees. I have fibromyalgia and starting in 2008, the pain in my legs was excruciating. I was losing my ability to walk. I shuffled along like a 95 year old, though I was only 47 at the time. I felt resigned that I would die very soon.

I was convinced I was not eating enough, but in fact my food record from the period shows I was eating eleven times a day. I ate cheap foods every day, thinking I was saving money. But what I was buying so cheaply was ill health. I was isolated emotionally and socially, and I had wild mood swings and rages. I believed in a benevolent God but was terrified to let her take control of my eating. I already walked with a cane, and I was about to get a walker or wheelchair.

Then a woman in another Twelve Step fellowship suggested I try a phone meeting of a ninety-day program, and I did. This program suggested I abstain from products made with sugar and flour. During one of my last stints in bed, I had bought a box of chocolates to reward myself for something. I said to myself, "I'll just eat five pieces to prove I have control over my eating." But half an hour after eating the chocolates, I felt the worst pain I had ever experienced. I finally made the connection: Sugar was killing me.

At another OA phone meeting I heard the term "abstinence." My friend from the other fellowship told me she had been abstinent for over twenty-two years. I realized that abstinence was a viable long-term lifestyle choice.

On December 10, 2008, I had my first full day of abstinence. I called into a meeting every day. I experienced a horrible withdrawal from sugar and flour, for which I'm thankful because I will think twice before going through that again. By the time I had been abstinent ten days, I'd lost my craving for sugar. This was a great mercy, because prior to becoming abstinent, I had a constant desire for sugar.

After thirty-five days of withdrawal I began to feel euphoria. I was on the pink cloud. The pain in my legs and body began to lessen. My mind had never been so clear and the depression miraculously lifted. I did Step One and admitted my total powerlessness. I did Step Two, deciding I believed that my Higher Power had the power to restore me to wholeness (sanity). And I affirmed that this Higher Power loved me enough and thought me worthy enough to restore me to sanity.

Then I surrendered my will to my Higher Power, along with my ideas about food that I'd been so sure were right. My recovery in OA has been about avoiding the foods and eating behaviors that were killing me, but also as part of the good self-care I'm learning to practice, I needed to eat those foods my medical nutritionist recommended to build myself up. My body was exhausted after years of abusing food.

By February 2009, after just two months of abstinence, all my physical pain was gone; I walked normally and threw away my cane. In the ensuing months, I walked briskly—a miracle! To date I have lost 120 pounds (54 kg), by the grace of God. When I rise in the morning, I say the Serenity Prayer and the Third, Seventh, and Eleventh Step prayers. I'm working on my Fourth Step and attending meetings daily. My home meeting is a midnight phone meeting.

By the way, I had gastric bypass surgery in the past. I lost very little weight after surgery because the problem was not in my stomach, it was in my head. I'm always going to be a compulsive overeater. I will continue to need to go to meetings, pray, do the Steps, help newcomers, work with a sponsor, write, and have an action plan. I'm grateful for that reality because OA has given me a new life.

I no longer think about death. I enjoy life and think about how to do God's will, how to be creative, and how to help someone else.

33

My Doctor Insisted

In May, 2006, at my doctor's insistence, I walked into my first OA meeting. I weighed 313 pounds (142 kg). I only wanted to show my doctor that this too wouldn't work and she would have to approve the bariatric surgery I wanted to save my life.

I had tried diet clubs, pills, and cognitive psychology, as well as every low-calorie and low-fat diet. All of them worked to some extent. In the end, though, they failed to stop my inexorable weight gain. If I lost weight, I only gained it back, and more.

I began overeating at puberty and became the chubby kid. When I bought clothes, I always had to go to the "husky" department. My peers began teasing me. I couldn't run very fast, so the kids nicknamed me "Speedy." That name stuck until we moved to Los Angeles in 1955. By then I had such low self-esteem that I avoided making new friends, got into fights, and was so shy I couldn't even talk to girls.

I started to diet and eventually lost a few pounds. I met the girl who would become my wife on a blind date in 1959. It was a blind date because I was too shy to ask her out directly. We married two years later, between my junior and senior year of college.

The stress of that senior year, with a pregnant wife and then a baby to take care of, plus a new job, caused me to really put on the pounds. It wasn't much later that I tipped the scales at more than 200 pounds (91 kg). Thus began my lifelong career of dieting, bingeing, gaining it all back, and dieting again, until, in the summer of 2002, I could no longer weigh myself on my bathroom scale.

I couldn't understand how I'd been able to lose weight successfully in the past but was now incapable of dieting more than a week at a time—usually not more than a day at a time. "Only one last time to the refrigerator and then I'll stop." Then, ten minutes later, I was back at the refrigerator looking for something more to eat. Or more frightening, as I lay in bed struggling to breathe, saying, "Please, God, tomorrow morning I'll start a diet." I wouldn't even make it past breakfast. "On Monday, I'll start." "Okay, then, on the first of the month." "Right after Thanksgiving... . Christmas... . New Year's Day."

And so it went until I visited my doctor's office in fall 2005. She took one look at my blood pressure and had me sit in a quiet room until my pressure went down, so she felt more confident I wouldn't have a stroke. She started me on cholesterol-lowering drugs, but a month later had to take me off because my liver was too fatty to tolerate them. She handed me a low-salt, low-fat diet and told me to go forth and lose weight. Yeah! Like that was all I needed. Like I haven't been on every diet imaginable in the past fifty-plus years.

But again, I started to diet. This time, I knew my life depended on it. I even lost a few pounds. But like all other diets I had ever been on, this diet too came to an end.

On Thanksgiving Day, 2005, a few chips with dip began a nonstop eating binge that didn't really end until May, 2006. This final binge erased all the progress I had made. I was desperate. I was ready to get my stomach stapled: the ultimate magic bullet. I knew the surgery could be dangerous, but I also knew if the surgery didn't work, I was a dead man anyway.

In early May, 2006, I begged my doctor to approve bariatric surgery. She said before she would approve the surgery, I had to see a therapist who specialized in eating disorders. The therapist said I had to agree to attend at least three OA meetings. That's how she saved my life.

On May 26, 2006, I walked into my first OA meeting. Only when I began working the Twelve Steps did I finally find the spiritual connection that allowed me not only to shed 150 pounds (68 kg) but also to begin my real recovery—and without the surgery.

I had my first spiritual awakening one year after the beginning of that last binge in 2005. My wife and I were driving to my daughter's home for Thanksgiving, 2006. My wife suddenly told me to take a shortcut rather than the direction I was headed. My first response was to shout, "Stop backseat driving." But before I could get the words out, a still, small voice in my head whispered, "Remember, you want to treat her with love, honor, dignity, and respect." So I thanked her and took the shortcut.

Wow! I thought. Where did that come from?

That evening was the best Thanksgiving I had ever had. I kept my abstinence. I ate reasonable portions, but when the desserts came out, I feared how I could handle them. Then that still, small voice in my head whispered, "Just say 'No thank you.'" And I did. Instead, I concentrated on enjoying my children and grandchildren and on the sheer joy of my abstinent life that day. I was surprised that I felt no anger at missing out on a favorite dish or dessert. I didn't feel deprived. I only felt profound gratitude for God's gifts to my family and me.

On the way home that evening, my wife started to complain about one of the guests. I started to join in when that still, small voice appeared again: "You asked to be relieved of the need to gossip; don't engage in it here." My mind raced. *This was the third time that night* I had heard from my Higher Power. That was my first real spiritual awakening. I began to accept that God was indeed listening to my prayers and was answering me, in his time and in his way. All I had to do was follow his will for me one day at a time. You see, I have pledged to follow his will for me with every fiber of my being. I pray daily only for knowledge of his will and the power and strength to carry it out. Why? Because my life, my health, and my sanity depend on it.

Thanks to my friends in OA, who share their lives with me; to my sponsor, who has become a personal friend; and to the grace of God; I have begun to really live my life, one day at a time.

34

FOOD IS NOT AN OPTION

One of my earliest memories is of sneaking into our back garden and eating the stale bread my mother had thrown out for the birds, an act unremarkable in itself. What remained with me are the feelings of calm and tranquility that came when the food hit my stomach. I remembered that and chased it through the first thirty-two years of my life to a dead end of misery.

My childhood was volatile, including the divorce of my parents, followed by the decline of my alcoholic mother, and the early exit of my father. A couple of stepfathers came and went. Unfortunately for my voracious appetite, money was tight and the food at home was rigorously healthy.

Looking back, I realize the situation stopped my weight from ballooning out of control, but nevertheless I was solid. I wanted to be slim and elegant like other girls at school; I didn't want lumpy fat over my hips. I didn't want to be stocky and thick. I wanted to feel feminine and attractive.

I tried to diet. I was full of resolve, bursting with desire to be slim. But I could never beat food. I watched friends push plates away with food left on them, and I genuinely couldn't understand how they did it. What was the secret? I could do it once, but I couldn't do it enough times to lose weight. Why was I the only one who was so useless?

Then I got my first part-time job—in a cafe. I worked there all summer and when school started again, I had no money to show for it, and I had gained 10 kilograms (22 lbs).

Around that time I heard about OA, and I decided to take a bulimic friend to a meeting. I went to support her, but I heard my story. I was excited, but I didn't like the name "Overeaters Anonymous," and besides, I was only 16. I was going to outrun this thing. I was never going to get as bad as these people. That night I heard there were certain foods that triggered compulsive eating. Sugar was that food for me. I also heard about eating to a food plan, so I took sugar away and ate only three meals a day. I did it like my life depended on it, and I lost weight. At last I had found something that could make an impact on my weight. A lightbulb went on.

But I couldn't stick to it. I was using OA like another diet: the "OA Do-It-Yourself Kit." The closest I could get to abstaining from compulsive eating was to have a few good days and then a blowout binge to let the pressure off. But I had lost weight and wasn't keen on gaining it back, so I started alternating junk food binges with fruit and vegetable binges to compensate.

I was getting a kick out of bingeing and not putting on weight. I started lengthening the fruit and vegetable binges. My weight was dropping, and I loved it. I couldn't think straight anymore, the girl who had gotten two scholarships in her final year of college. I didn't care. My hair was dropping out. My skin was so dry; I felt like an old lady. I was depressed and wanted to be apart from people because I couldn't keep up the "happy person" image very long. But I held on to being thin: If I was thin, then I didn't have a problem with food. I was in control. And if I was thin, I wasn't the same me who had felt so unlikable as a chubby kid.

Years passed and nothing changed. I was living in London, where my degree had secured me a job my brain could no longer handle. My body was suffering from nutrient deprivation. I was around 43 kilograms (95 lbs).

I returned to New Zealand. Being thin now felt like a booby prize. I had food and could eat what I wanted when I wanted, but I had lost access to the rest of my life as a consequence.

I tried to sort myself out through therapy. After two years I finally said, "There's this thing I do with food… ." I explained the bingeing and asked my therapist if it could have anything to do with the way I felt. Her answer hit me like a punch in the gut. She said, "Nothing will change for you until you do something about your problem with food." I was ready to change.

I went back to OA on March 14, 2005. I was 32 years old. I have been abstinent since that date, for which I am overwhelmingly grateful. I was willing to do anything to feel better. I knew OA worked. I hadn't wanted it before, but I sure wanted it now.

Whatever the other members said worked for them, I did. They said they had sponsors. I got one. They said they made a food plan and stuck to it. So did I. They said they went to plenty of meetings. I went to plenty. They said they shared. I shared. They said they did service. I did service. They said they did the Steps. I did the Steps. They said they got a Higher Power that made sense to them, and they used it. I used mine.

The first few months of abstinence were like riding a bucking bronco—I held on for dear life to the reins of OA while my emotions kicked and bucked. Then things calmed down and slowly started getting better.

Now, seven years later, I still do the things that got me abstinent. OA has taught me that by continually working the Steps, Tools, and Traditions, I can keep adding skills to the basics that got me abstinent. Each skill I learn helps my life work better and makes my emotions easier to manage. Each one makes me feel better about myself and makes my relationships go more smoothly. What am I really saying? These skills make me more comfortable in the world, more able to cope with the situations that life constantly throws me. The result is I feel content with myself and my life. That is an enormous change for me.

The better I feel, the more able I am to tackle dreams, large and small, that I previously never had the inner resources to attempt. Because I am not using food anymore, I learn from all these new experiences. I can look people in the eye now. It's a life of dignity.

As a result of sticking around and doing the suggested things in this program, I am able to eat my planned meals, enjoy them, and not crave food in between. I have been able to keep my marriage to my dear husband, whom I love very much. I've been able to begin a career I had always dreamed about but was never able to start. I've been able to regain my physical health and give birth to a beautiful son who has never seen me in that other life. And I pray, with OA's help, he never will.

35

THE TINY ACORN GROWS INTO
A MIGHTY OAK

When I came to OA in 1995, I had three years of sobriety with alcohol and drugs. I was 70 to 80 pounds (32 to 36 kg) overweight and had suffered a heart attack in May 1994. I was 36 years old.

My health was devastated by bad genes and years of bingeing on alcohol, drugs, sex, cigarettes, and most of all, food. After an emergency angioplasty, doctors told me I had three major blockages in the arteries surrounding my heart and was lucky to be alive: "You are our youngest patient with arteriosclerosis; what are you doing to yourself?" I felt like the whole universe was pointing at me and sneering.

I was overwhelmed with a toxic load of shame that I had tried desperately to escape for years: shame for being gay; for being fat, short and bald; for my alcoholic father's suicide when I was 7. I had suffered the trauma of my mother's death from a heart attack when I was in college, and I felt unbearable shame about humiliating sexual abuse I experienced from an obese member of the clergy when I was 12. To numb the shame, my solution had always been to binge on donuts and chocolate cake until I was sick.

It took me several years in OA to grasp the idea of food addiction. I tried in vain to transfer my sobriety from alcohol and drugs to abstinence with food. Unfortunately, at that time there were only a few abstinent people in the OA meetings in my area. Many of the longtimers were still obese and living in the disease.

I unsuccessfully tried three weeks at an expensive treatment center, but I started to realize that I needed someone to help me understand the Steps and Tools of Overeaters Anonymous. A friend took me to an OA group that stressed abstaining from sugar, flour, and volume, and weighing and measuring portions. I found a sponsor who helped me devise a food plan appropriate to my needs. I began to use the OA Tools every day, and I called my sponsor to give him my food plan each morning. Miraculously, I let go of my compulsive need to control my food and weight, and I concentrated on working the program by attending meetings and doing service. Within months, my weight and blood lipids were at healthful numbers. My cardiologists were finally happy.

Once I had some physical recovery, I began to look at the intense resentment I felt toward organized religion. I equated God with the crazy and abusive adults from my childhood, and I allowed myself to be a victim. I am a horticulturist, and one of my sponsors, who is a gardener, suggested that I look to nature for my Higher Power.

"A tiny acorn grows into a mighty oak," he would tell me as we did Step work in his lush greenhouse in the middle of winter. Slowly I began to understand the Second Step, which my sponsor referred to as the roadmap to the following ten Steps.

In writing Fourth Step inventories, I started to examine my emotionally dependent relationship with my partner. He was a professor I had begun an affair with at college. I met him when I was 20 and he was 43; we were together for twenty-five years. He was rich, successful, and famous in his field, and I jumped on for the ride. It made me feel important, but in reality I was losing myself in the process of hiding in his shadow. I allowed the terror I felt about this relationship to lure me back to the food, and by the fall of 2001; I was in relapse.

In 2002, one of my nieces died of anorexia nervosa. I hadn't seen her for several years and had no idea she was suffering from this disease. I was as devastated as someone numb on food can possibly be.

That fall, a program friend hysterically confessed to me that he and my partner were having an affair. In my extreme codependency, I focused on calming him down, and then I ordered a pizza. My life felt so out of control, food was the only thing that made sense to me.

I began a compulsive period of trying to fix myself by going to treatment centers and therapists, but the weight came back, and once again, I was eating until I was sick. I had purged and restricted food in high school and college. Terrifyingly, those two forms of the addiction began to look attractive again. I would have a month of abstinence and then binge; a few weeks and then binge; a day and then binge. My compulsion to drink began to return.

The desperation I felt in relapse forced me to work a much deeper, more sincere program. Every morning I got down on my knees and did the first three Steps, begging God for surrender, which I now believe is a divine gift. When I binged, OA members told me to "keep coming back" no matter what. They said it so many times I got sick of hearing it. But they loved me when I hated myself, and they often reminded me that, "The only requirement for OA membership is a desire to stop eating compulsively" (Tradition Three). The literature told me to pray for the willingness and ability to work my food program each day and to thank God each night, even if I binged that day.

Abstinent members opened several new meetings in my area, where I learned more about the OA Twelve Steps and Twelve Traditions and how our Fellowship worked. OA became my life raft, and I hung on with all the perseverance I could muster.

My Higher Power gave me the gift of abstinence in the summer of 2005, and I have been given a daily reprieve ever since. I've learned to watch the OA longtimers who have what I want, and I try to do what they do. I come to meetings and share honestly, doing my best to let go of my ego's desire to sound like I have it all together.

I talk to my sponsor each day, and I am guiding several sponsees through the Steps.

Today I am at a healthful weight of 155 pounds (70 kg), and I ask God daily for the willingness and ability to follow a heart-friendly food and exercise plan. I am a responsible, single, abstinent adult who choses today to live in the solution of Overeaters Anonymous.

36

SEVENTY-FIVE AND FULLY ALIVE

I came to my first Overeaters Anonymous meeting in October 1974 at age 37. After many years of successful dieting followed by more weight gain, I was excited by what I heard at this meeting. I heard the good news that I have a disease and I'm not alone; many others also suffer with this malady. The other good news was that the solution is found in the Twelve Steps of recovery. I knew this was an answer to my prayers because I had asked God to help me with my food problem, and God sent an angel who told me about the meeting.

I made a feeble attempt to work the Steps without the help of a sponsor. My program consisted of attending a meeting once a week and doing service in my group. It worked for a while, and I even lost weight. I used the food plan given out at that time, but I would slip back into eating the foods that caused my cravings and wonder why I couldn't stay abstinent. I said I was growing emotionally and spiritually. This was a lie I told myself; the only thing growing was my body. I did this for twelve years and then fell into relapse and ate for the next five years.

I never left the program, but I didn't attend strong meetings because I felt shame and didn't want to be accountable to those who were working the program. I became more isolated, and I felt guilty about being around the program for so many years and still not getting it. As my disease progressed, I became more and more focused on my next binge. It became more important than family and friends. The binge brought temporary relief from pain but destroyed everything that was important in my life.

In December 1991, I reached an all-time low. I was 65 pounds (29 kg) overweight and bingeing daily. My physical health began to suffer. Emotionally, I was full of fear and resentment and felt I would be better off dead. I was extremely self-centered and hurt a lot of people if things didn't go my way. I was spiritually dead and was trying to fill a hole inside of me with food. I slumped to my knees crying out to my Higher Power to help me.

On January 2, 1992, I attended a strong meeting where many long-time abstainers welcomed me with open arms. On that day I made a decision that would change my life. I committed a food plan to a sponsor and began to work the Steps of the program.

What have these years of experience taught me? They taught me that I have to be completely honest with others and myself. I couldn't stop eating until I admitted to my innermost self that I am a compulsive overeater, and I couldn't get help until I recognized the need for help. I needed to admit to my trigger foods and get on a plan of eating that would clear my brain, so I could be open to working the Steps with a sponsor.

The most important thing I've learned is that depending on a Higher Power of my understanding, whom I call God, would change me. As the result of depending on God and working the Steps, I have been continuously abstinent since January 2, 1992, and my obsession with food has been removed. I wanted to be thin all my life, and I got my wish. I lost 65 pounds (29 kg), and I have maintained a healthy body weight. I am a 75-year-old female who has normal blood pressure and good cholesterol and takes only one prescription medication.

I have the Fellowship of Overeaters Anonymous I can count on for direction, support, affirmation, and love. I have a life I never could have imagined twenty years ago. When I was eating, I was a shy, introverted, fearful person. Today I can look people in the eye and not be afraid. By working the Steps daily I have been able to take an honest look at myself and admit to what needs to be changed in me, not what needs to be changed in everyone else. As a result, my relationships have improved. I do not need to be right anymore.

I have gotten to do service at all OA levels, which has enhanced my program and helped me to grow as a person. Service has taken me out of myself and opened me up to others. It has given me an interest in OA as a whole and furthered my understanding of how important the Twelve Traditions and Twelve Concepts are to OA unity. I have even found out how the Traditions can be applied to my personal life.

I was instrumental in starting an intergroup in my area. I served on the region board after being a region representative, and then I served on the Board of Trustees after being a delegate at the World Service Business Conference. I have come to care about what is going on in OA and am happy to be part of making decisions that affect OA as a whole. There is no way I could have done all this without the help of my Higher Power.

The last twenty years have been amazing. I turned my will and life over to a God I didn't fully understand; I told someone my deepest, darkest secrets; I looked at my character defects; and I made amends. The most amazing part has been developing a relationship with a God of my understanding. Quiet times of prayer and meditation are absolutely necessary to my continued recovery. By spending time with God each day, I become more the person God wants me to be—loving, tolerant, patient, and kind. The Twelve Steps have brought me to God in a way I never could have imagined.

It took me many years to get where I am today, but I am evidence that long-term recovery after relapse is possible. I don't believe God wants me to destroy myself with food. I pray daily that I never take that destructive path again. My life depends on it. My disease is in remission as long as I abstain and work the Steps of the program. If the miracle happened to me, it can happen to anyone who wants it.

37

No Longer a Little Girl

My disease has manifested in every form. I've been an overweight, compulsive overeater; a starving anorexic; and an obsessive bulimic. My issues with food and body image started in childhood. Some of my earliest and most vivid memories deal with the shame I felt around my body and my eating.

One night when I was 5 years old, my sister and I were getting ready for bed. I took off my clothes to put on pajamas. She looked at my body and said, "You're fat." I burst into tears and ran to my mother, looking for comfort.

"She called me fat!" I choked out through tears.

My mother's lips tightened into a thin line. "Put on a shirt and she won't be able to see you," she replied curtly.

That was the message I received as a child: My body and my eating were things to be covered up, hidden, ashamed of.

At the dinner table a few years later, my father watched me eat my meal and exclaimed with disgust, "You're like a human vacuum cleaner!" I was mortified and crushed. I locked myself in my room and cried myself to sleep. Over the next seven years, I continued to eat to soothe myself. Food comforted me when my parents did not.

When I was 15, my mother took me shopping for school clothes. In the dressing room, I could see the disappointment in my mother's face. Not one single item in the trendy juniors' section fit me. I wept silently in the car on the way home as I listened to my mother tell me how much easier my life would be if I were thin. I weighed 196 pounds (89 kg).

I was so desperate to lose weight, I began starving myself. The same way food had comforted me in childhood, anorexia comforted me in my teens. I would eat a miniscule amount of food at breakfast and lunch just to stay conscious during school, then I would make excuses to skip dinner every night. If I had to eat, I would make up for it by exercising until I couldn't move. My parents readily accepted this behavior for nearly two years, and they were incredibly pleased that I was losing weight. After I had lost 35 pounds (16 kg), they no longer looked at me with disappointment.

I moved away and started college at age 17. While there, I found that I was too weak-willed to maintain my anorexia. There were too many parties and social gatherings involving food. In my freshman year I gained back 10 pounds (5 kg). Then I turned to the behavior that would quickly consume me: bulimia. The first time I purged after a big meal, I thought it was a onetime thing. I was so wrong.

I am still astounded by how rapidly bulimia took over my life. In a matter of weeks, I was purging everything I ate without exception. I spent the next three years with my head in toilets and trash cans, violently vomiting the massive amounts of food I stuffed into my body. At the time, I worked in a grocery store (big mistake), and I stole food from work every night. I stole food from roommates. I was moody and lied constantly. Physically, I was in bad shape. My back teeth rotted. I was frequently dizzy and fainted occasionally. I had constant pain in my head, neck, and chest. My weight was down to an all-time low, and I was weak.

During the peak (or rather, the low) point of my bulimia a friend asked me to give her a ride somewhere. I picked her up, and as soon as she buckled her seat belt, she turned to look at me. "I need to talk to you about something serious," she said. "I think you're bulimic and I want you to get help." I was stunned. She had caught me so off guard that I couldn't deny it. Bulimia was my big secret. I thought I had hidden it so well! Apparently not.

That friend saved my life. After that car ride, I started seeing a therapist, and a year after that, I walked into my first OA meeting. I was 19 years old.

I considered myself an atheist at the time, and I was skeptical about a bunch of people who sat in a circle holding hands and praying to God. But I met people in that first meeting who knew what I was going through because they had gone through the same things themselves. I met people who drove to the grocery store in the middle of the night to buy food they knew they were going to throw up later. Most important, I met people who were free of these things. It was unbelievable to me. I didn't yet believe in the program, but I couldn't deny that these people had something I wanted. I kept coming back.

Some people come into OA and are "struck abstinent" at their first meeting. I was not. It took a full year for me to surrender to the program, get abstinent from bingeing and purging, find a sponsor, and start working the Twelve Steps. Now I see I needed that year for my fear to melt away. I was afraid of what life would be like without compulsive eating. After that year, I became totally willing to make abstinence the most important thing in my life without exception.

When I got abstinent, my program was very rigid. I planned my food and turned it over to a sponsor every day. I wrote a Tenth Step every night. I went to three meetings a week and sponsored three OA members.

Recently my sponsor pointed out that I was getting compulsive about the rigidity of my program; I had begun to make the planning and the structure my Higher Power. She was right. Since then, I have been working my program around one major concept: God will take care of me. I have let go of control and truly turned my food and my life over to God. This has freed me. I still maintain the daily aspects of my program, but now I do it on God's time, not on my time.

I believe strongly in the Twelve Steps. Working the Steps helped me unearth everything I had learned to keep hidden over the years. I believe the Steps can be summed up in three basic principles: Trust in God, Clean House, and Do for Others. Living my life around these principles has allowed me to live through uncomfortable moments, instead of hiding from them behind piles of food. I stay honest even in difficult moments, and I give service to others.

I am no longer the little girl seeking comfort in all the wrong places. I now seek comfort in only two places—the Fellowship of Overeaters Anonymous and God. I know I will be taken care of.

38

LONER FINDS A HOME

On Thanksgiving I ate my third heaping plateful, looked at the person beside me, and realized I would be her weight in three months. For the past six months, every month, I had put on 25 pounds (11 kg) the first two weeks and taken off 20 pounds (9 kg) the last two weeks. Feeling I could no longer stop for the last two weeks, I knew I would put on 50 pounds (23 kg) per month, and this would continue, I figured, until I exploded.

At home that evening, I looked at meeting information a friend had given me. I decided to try OA that Sunday afternoon. I went and hated it, grabbed brochures and a meeting list, pigged out all week, then went to a different meeting. There, a woman approached me and told me to call her the next morning, starting me off on the road of happy destiny. I have never binged again. I recently celebrated thirty-one years of abstinent recovery offered by the Twelve Steps of Overeaters Anonymous. What happened in between?

For three years, I called my sponsor daily, attended two to six meetings a week, attended retreats, and did whatever my sponsor suggested. At a Big Book study weekend, led by an AA member who had been sober thirty-four years, I knew I never wanted to overeat again. So I followed the directions in *Alcoholics Anonymous* step by step, under the guidance of my abstinent and sane sponsor. I completed the first nine Steps in eighteen months and have never looked back. My sponsor's assurance that a Step thoroughly taken would be done once and for all has proven true for me. The first nine Steps provide a solid foundation upon which I live today, working Steps Ten, Eleven, and Twelve regularly.

When I got married, I spent the morning of my wedding day with my sponsor, clearing away some resentments and fears that had built up. With no wedding cake because I don't eat sugar and no champagne because I don't drink alcohol, the wedding was the best ever! I ate my weighed-and-measured meal, and food was not an issue.

At three years abstinent, my husband and I moved to rural South Africa for six years. As there were no OA meetings near me and I did not speak the local language, I went to open AA meetings in English when I could—difficult without a phone or car—and exchanged letters with my sponsor in the United States and other OA members. Annual trips by airplane to the nearest OA meetings helped; local members hosted me in their homes. I depended upon *Lifeline* and OA audio recordings and used *Alcoholics Anonymous* for a reminder of how to live this program each day. My service to OA was in the form of daily abstinence, letters to *Lifeline,* and sharing the message with people I met. I got a lifetime subscription to *Lifeline* when it was being offered, so I always had a new copy to pass on to anyone who expressed interest in OA.

I learned to use AA when OA was not available. I subscribed to an AA loners newsletter published in South Africa. I realized OA could be self-supporting in this area, so I started OAsis, an "OA Loners Meeting in Print." I invited other loners I'd met through OA to join the meeting in print. Watching this meeting grow to include more than one hundred people around the world and become a registered OA meeting was a privilege. It continued for more than a decade, into the late 1990s, until electronic options entered the scene.

I learned lots of helpful lessons from my first sponsor. The first was never to use distance or timing as an excuse not to get to a meeting. When I lived in English-speaking countries, I visited the nearest OA meetings while checking out affordable venues to start a meeting within 10 minutes from my home. I never wanted to have the excuse that my home meeting was too far away or I couldn't get there in bad weather. I found a venue I could afford even if no one else showed up, that was accessible in a snowstorm, and that was at a time that worked for me. I registered with the World Service Office and the intergroup, advertised in local newspapers, posted signs, and showed up. If no one came, I still followed the entire format, "listened" to a speaker from *Lifeline,* then wrote a share and posted it to *Lifeline.* I was just grateful to have a meeting and to have been available for a newcomer who might have arrived at any time.

Another lesson I learned was not to overeat no matter what. That means I may have to drive two hours to a meeting, make fifteen phone calls if a resentment is burning me up, or take my packed dinner to a fancy event. For me, the most important thing in my life without exception is abstinence. I will do anything to keep it. My children, who are now 27 and 24 years old, grew up knowing I do not share my food; I do not toast in the New Year; I do not bake birthday cakes. But they also know I love them and try to be the best Mum I can be. When I make a mistake or mistreat them, they know I always make an apology before the day is over.

Pregnancy in OA was amazing! Abstinence means that I provide my body with the fuel it needs. As doctors informed me of new needs, I worked with my sponsor to make necessary changes to my food plan. During the worst of labor, I focused on a stitchery of the Serenity Prayer, improving my conscious contact with a Higher Power with each breath. Taking this program one day at a time, one minute at a time, means I can face any situation with sanity, knowing that I am in the care of a Higher Power. What an amazing way to live!

Another lesson I learned from my sponsor is to always have a sponsor. When my first sponsor went back to the food, I had a new temporary sponsor before the day was out. When I travel for business or pleasure, I get a temporary sponsor where I am staying, often just for a few days. When I move, I find a local sponsor who is abstinent; working Steps Ten, Eleven, and Twelve; and available around the clock.

I had my second sponsor for sixteen years. During those years, when I lived in other countries, I had a local sponsor too, sometimes from AA because no one in OA was abstinent and working the Steps. The AA person wasn't a compulsive overeater, so our problems were with different substances, but we shared a common solution—working the Twelve Steps of recovery.

I am grateful for my physical, mental, and spiritual recovery. Someone once told me this simple program boils down to saying please in the morning and thank you at night, and using the time in between to help the person still suffering from compulsive overeating. That's been working for me all these years.

I look forward to being in OA; working Steps Ten, Eleven, and Twelve; and living free of the compulsion for the rest of my life, one day at a time!

39

A BAD CASE OF DENIAL

I didn't get help with my food until three years after my second open-heart surgery and a doctor telling me I was dying. My doctor must have told me this many times before; I was 100 pounds (45 kg) overweight. Somehow, the thought of dying did not penetrate my consciousness despite overwhelming evidence of chronic heart disease. My doctor's fear for me lifted my denial. When I left my cardiologist's office, I really thought I could go home and stop. Tomorrow was today.

After an abstinent dinner that night, I found myself with my head in a bag of one of my favorite binge foods in less than an hour. I could not stop. But there was no more denial. I knew I was killing myself despite having a wonderful family and the job of my dreams. This reality, which I call the gift of desperation, led to clinical depression. My cardiologist sent me to a therapist, and the therapist gave me a choice: drugs for depression or OA. I chose OA. That was close to twenty-three years ago.

The longest ride of my life was the ride to my first meeting, which I still remember well. For years I had rationalized that I would start my diet tomorrow. One more day wouldn't matter. Prior to that rationalization, I yo-yo dieted for many years.

After my first open-heart surgery at age 37, I lost all my excess weight, more than 60 pounds (27 kg). A year later, it was all back. Eight years later at 45, I had my second open-heart surgery. The operation was not accompanied by weight loss this time around, just rationalizations. Three years later, I went to my first OA meeting. The last time I got on the scale I was 246 pounds (111 kg). Then I just stopped weighing. I presently weigh 162 pounds (73 kg) and with God's help have stayed within a 5-pound (2-kg) range ever since losing the weight, which took close to a year.

That first OA meeting was a miracle. OA members talked about food just like I felt about food. They were powerless too, but they were laughing and thin, and I was crying and dying. For the first time in months, I felt that I might live. I had hope. But it wasn't quite that easy.

My first surrender was to find a sponsor and do what he told me to do. My sponsor told me he knew I was powerless over food and could not stop eating compulsively. But I could (1) agree to a food plan free of binge or trigger foods; (2) call before that first bite, which meant eating anything beyond what was on my food plan; and (3) if that failed, I could call after taking that first compulsive bite. My sponsor told me to call in my daily food plan choices every morning, which I did for two years.

Finally, my ego helped me. I was too embarrassed to call in slips, so I always called before my first bite. And he always talked me down off the cliff. One night, after an extensive discussion, he told me to hang up the phone and run upstairs to bed. It worked. I would tell him I was hungry, angry, lonely, and tired. He would say, "Wonderful. That's just where you are supposed to be. You are feeling your feelings." This gave me the courage to walk through the fear and come out the other side. I learned that feelings are not reality.

After three months detoxing from the food, I tackled Steps Four and Five and a lot more feelings. I learned I was motivated by fear. My sponsor gave me a list of one hundred and two defects. I had to list the underlying reason for these defects, which I realized was always fear. My fears included economic insecurity, rejection, and failure. And fear was essentially a lack of trust in a Higher Power.

I was always afraid I wasn't good enough; I was a failure despite how much I might accomplish. And I had always numbed this feeling with food, not recognizing what I was doing. Slowly I began to trust. Not eating compulsively was a miracle I could only attribute to a Higher Power whom I now call God. I could trust my sponsor was sent from HP to help me. And I trusted my fellow members, who showed me unconditional love by telling me about their fears and journey through the food wars.

With guidance from my sponsor, I was able to give these defects and fears to God in Steps Six and Seven and get right with the world by making amends in Steps Eight and Nine. My relationship with God and others grew day by day as I journeyed through the Steps. Step Four of the AA *Twelve and Twelve,* which was the literature available to us twenty-two years ago, indicates "our total inability to form a true partnership with another human being" (p. 53). Steps Four through Nine have helped me form such relationships. Steps Two and Three helped me form a relationship with God. And Step One brought me to my knees to start the journey. Either surrender or die. I surrendered, and I have a life beyond my wildest dreams. The promises of the program have all come true for me. I have a relationship with my brother, whom I hadn't talk to for the better part of twenty years, and I can look any man in the eye without feeling shame.

Many miracles beyond the food have occurred in my life, not the least of which is being alive. My first bypass graft is close to thirty-four years old. Fifty percent of grafts break down in the first ten years. The last repair wasn't supposed to keep me going more than two to three years. That was five years ago!

But to my ongoing amazement, denial always lurks around the corner. Two years into program, I missed meetings for two weeks while on vacation and thought I was "normal." I didn't eat but came close. I committed then and there to doing Steps Ten, Eleven, and

Twelve every single day for the rest of my life as maintenance.

I read pages 86 to 88 of the Big Book (*Alcoholics Anonymous*, 4th ed.) every day, which give questions to facilitate a daily inventory of myself and help me focus on what God wants me to do. I also read OA's "Just For Today" card, which helps me focus on positive things to do for God. I read four daily readers, including OA's and my church's, to enhance my connection with HP.

My way, self-will, got me here. God's way, Step Twelve, keeps me serene and free of my compulsion to overeat.

40

NO MORE STORE HOPPING

Never in a million years did I think I would be able to stop bingeing and purging, compulsively exercising and starving. Nor did I hope that I could have a normal life like people I envied because they could eat one of something or stop eating when (or even before!) they were full.

But by the grace of God and Overeaters Anonymous, I have been freed from the compulsion with food since April 1981; have maintained a healthy, thin weight; and get to experience life on life's terms without having to use food to numb the feelings.

I was born a compulsive overeater. I don't remember a single day in my life that I was not obsessed with food, eating, or the size of my body. My parents' relationship was full of angry fights, and my father was violent with my mother, my three siblings, and me. The only comfort I found was in food, and I always ate until I was stuffed. I was an active kid, so I didn't become super overweight, but as my disease of selfishness and self-centeredness progressed so did my food consumption and weight.

When I turned 13, I decided to go on a diet because I was entering high school and wanted to be thin. I weighed about 140 pounds (63 kg). I read in a magazine about anorexia and bulimia, which were not well-known in 1973, and I thought, "Wow, why didn't I think of that?"

I lost 30 pounds (14 kg) over the summer by starving, running, and throwing up after every meal. At last I had arrived! I would be popular, get a boyfriend, get straight As, and be the homecoming queen. But first, I had to lose just 5 more pounds (2 kg), then 5 more, then 5 more. By Christmas I was down to 97 pounds (44 kg) at five feet four inches (162 cm) tall, and I stayed there for about ten minutes. When no boyfriend came knocking on my door and I got straight Bs and no nomination for anything, I thought, "Why am I working so hard? I'm not getting all those magic things that happen to thin people. I might as well eat." In one month I gained 30 pounds (14 kg), but I didn't stop there. By the end of that school year, I weighed more than 175 pounds (80 kg).

Then started all the fad diets, gimmicks, and self-help book ideas. I gained 10 pounds (5 kg) during my hypnosis class in which the teacher told me to imagine my binge foods covered in worms. The next week, my classmates said how well that worked and how they were able to stop eating those foods. I gained 5 pounds (2 kg) that week.

I began stealing food to support my habit. I worked at fast-food places but had to quit when I outgrew the largest sized uniform. I ate everything but the baby when babysitting; went store hopping in bad neighborhoods with an unreliable car; and didn't care about anything but food, eating, and throwing up. I was suicidal and homicidal and didn't care if I lived or died. I had hit bottom.

One day my mom told me about a neighbor who had been obese and lost 125 pounds (57 kg) through OA. I grabbed the phone and called. I was 17 years old. I went to a meeting and knew immediately that I was home. Even though it took me three years to get abstinent, and I hit new bottoms I didn't know were possible, I did one thing right. I kept coming back. Although I was wiping crumbs off my face when walking through the door, I never stopped coming to meetings and calling my sponsor.

My recovery began when I took Step One and conceded to my innermost self that I am a compulsive overeater. I have lost the ability to control my food and will never get it back. As long as I don't let my denial take over and start to think I can eat certain foods in moderation or at random without consequence, I will continue to be abstinent. Sometimes I hear newcomers lament, "I don't think I can go the rest of my life without eating cookies or cupcakes." And I'm thinking, "Please God, let me go the rest of my life without eating cookies or cupcakes because those foods will kill me." And by the grace of God, the compulsion for eating food not on my food plan has been lifted, one day at a time. I am free from compulsion and not obsessed with food, food plans, or my body.

In thirty years of recovery, I have put myself through college; launched a successful career; married; bought a house; had a baby; divorced; told my father I loved him moments before he died; traveled to Europe three times; rode my bike more than ten thousand miles in four years; had my beloved dog of fourteen years die in my arms; made financial amends to all the stores and restaurants from which I stole merchandise and food; and many other things.

I live my life free of fear because I have a loving God guiding me. In my daily prayer and meditation, I remind myself that I turned my will and life over to my Higher Power one day back in 1982 when I worked the Third Step with my sponsor. I reaffirm daily that I surrender to my Higher Power and ask for help in finding and doing God's will for that twenty-four hours.

I have every reason to have hope today. Miracles continue to happen in my life. That doesn't mean I get what I want and magic fairy dust is sprinkled over me. It does mean I have a program and Tools that will get me through everything life offers without having to numb out or kill myself with food.

Thank you, Overeaters Anonymous. Thank you to everyone who comes to meetings, shares, sponsors, does service, abstains, helps newcomers, and keeps coming back. You gave me my life back, and I am forever grateful.

41

FROM ANGRY TEEN TO SERENE MOM

I walked into my first meeting of Overeaters Anonymous four days before my 18th birthday. I don't remember what was said at that first meeting, but I do remember the feeling of being in the right place. I heard people talk about food and the unmanageability of their lives in a way that I related to intensely.

When people ask how I came to program so young and stayed, I can only say I stayed because nothing in my life was working. I didn't have much weight to lose, maybe 10 or 15 pounds, but food ruled my life. Out of control bingeing and intense body obsession drove me to constant attempts to diet and exercise.

At first I wasn't sure if OA would work for me because of the "God thing." My family scoffed at religion and never discussed spirituality. So the word God was almost enough to make me turn around and walk out. Lucky for me, my life was a mess. I could not point to anything and say, "See, that part of my life is working, so I must not be that bad." I hated my body; couldn't stop eating compulsively; had no friends or boyfriend; was mean and nasty to my family; and was full of fear, resentment, and self-pity.

So I stuck around in spite of my fears about God. I raised all the usual questions about a Higher Power such as, "How could God exist when there is war, child abuse, and kids who die of cancer?" People told me I didn't have to wrestle with those questions; I could lay them aside and seek a Higher Power of my understanding, whatever that might mean. No one told me I had to believe in a certain God.

The other suggestion people made was that I "act as if." One day, desperate in the face of the food, I did just that. I got down on my knees and said my first prayer, "God, I don't know what you are, or if you're even out there; but if you're there, please help me because I can't stop eating compulsively." I got up from my knees and was abstinent for two weeks from that day, which had been impossible before. I still wasn't sure what this Higher Power was, but something inside cracked open enough to allow me to consider it. That was my first spiritual experience.

In spite of this, I continued to have a lot of trouble with food for my first four months in program. I had brief periods of not eating compulsively but couldn't maintain abstinence. Then one night at work, I felt the overwhelming compulsion to eat. I was a restaurant hostess and couldn't leave my post to make a phone call, so I prayed instead. I didn't just ask for help. I said, "I trust you, God. I can't do this, but I know you can. Please help me."

I said this prayer over and over for the rest of my shift. When my shift ended, I made a program call, went home, had an abstinent dinner, and went to bed. On that day, I went from white-knuckling to being graced with the ability to abstain.

I had an initial pink-cloud abstinence but didn't work the Steps. I started them but never stuck with a sponsor. Each time I changed sponsors, I went back to Step One. In spite of surrendering the food, I never got past Step Three, so my emotional and spiritual disease persisted.

Then I hit a new bottom. I had been abstinent for a year and a half, yet I was still miserable and lonely. Someone said to me, "You know, the Steps work for that." Of course I had heard people talk about the Steps, but that day I really *heard* it. Not long after, I shared at a meeting that I wanted to work the Steps and was looking for a sponsor. A woman who said she couldn't sponsor me long-term offered to start working the Steps with me right away. She got me started on my Fourth Step and saved my life.

The Steps turned out to be what I needed all along: a way to change on the inside. I believe that if I had continued as I was, following a food plan but not doing the Step work necessary for inner change, I would have eaten compulsively again.

The Fourth Step was a turning point in my recovery because for the first time I was able to take responsibility. Working the Fourth Step and giving it away in the Fifth Step, I started to see my part, the ways in which my own actions and fears had added to the mess in my life. I began to see that I didn't have to be a victim.

My spiritual recovery began when I opened myself to the idea of a Higher Power. My physical recovery began when I took the first three Steps around food and was graced with abstinence. The Fourth and Fifth Steps began my true, emotional recovery.

Over the years, as I continued to abstain and work the Steps, my life got better. I grew up in program—falling in love for the first time, getting my heart broken, staying up late dancing, earning my bachelor's degree, and mending my relationship with my mother through working the Ninth Step. I was relieved of the horrible body obsession that had plagued me since I was 10. I fell in love again, used the program Tools to nurture that relationship, and was married.

When I had been abstinent for ten years, I was diagnosed with Crohn's disease, a chronic autoimmune disorder. The diagnosis was a huge blow. I was scared, sad, and angry with my body and my Higher Power. I had many conversations, crying with my sponsor. This was the beginning of a change in my faith.

For my first decade in OA, just as people had suggested, I had laid aside those big questions about how God could coexist with all the pain in the world and instead focused on developing a personal relationship with a Higher Power. But now I faced a dilemma: If I believed in a God that brought good things into my life, did that mean God was also responsible for the bad things? And how could I trust that Higher Power? My health crisis opened the doors for all the larger questions about pain and suffering, which I could no longer ignore.

I continued to pray, although I didn't know to what. As I talked about Higher Power with others who identified as agnostic or atheist, read program literature written from those perspectives, and continued with my own Step work, a new conception of Higher Power came into my life, one that works for me today. I consider myself agnostic. I no longer believe in a God that controls things, because I simply cannot reconcile the pain and suffering in the world with the idea of an omnipotent, loving God.

I do believe there is a spiritual force in the universe, which I can tap into for help, although I don't know exactly what this power is. I used to feel the need to define my Higher Power. Today I find the most peace in *not* trying to define it. I recognize many powers greater than myself—nature, life, and death to name a few—and that my life is saner when I surrender than when I try to fight them. I also think the Steps are a Power greater than myself.

Overeaters Anonymous has given me a life when once I was just managing to survive. I have been abstinent now for seventeen years, nearly half my life. I maintain a healthy weight and feel comfortable in my own skin. As I write these words, I am in the final weeks of my second, abstinent pregnancy. I am grateful to have gained only a healthy amount of weight with each pregnancy and have been able to experience both the joys and fears of pregnancy without the haze of food taking over.

Today I have a home group that I attend every week. I also attend a monthly special focus meeting for moms in OA. I try to always have one service position at the meeting level. I have two sponsees, and I get a lot out of hearing them work the Steps. I have a sponsor and am going through the Steps again, because I know there is always more work to do. I follow a food plan that works for me. I read program literature every morning to help get my head on straight. I pray every morning, asking for help with my food and my life, and I say a prayer of thanks in the evening.

I am grateful for my life and my abstinence, and to all of you, walking the road of recovery with me.

APPENDICES

APPENDIX A

The Role of a Plan of Eating in Recovery from Compulsive Eating

I've been in practice as a registered dietitian for thirty-three years. I first became interested in obesity and weight management when I began my master's program; I wrote my thesis on the factors that influence success in weight loss programs. I found that success required a strong program of recovery and a special, supportive friend. I did not realize I was describing Overeaters Anonymous until years afterward.

I worked for years in hospitals and weight loss programs. What I learned in my training worked well for some people but not at all for others. When I heard the concept of food as part of an addictive process, I knew immediately it was the key I had been seeking.

I believe that people can be addicted to food, and it's important for them to identify and remove from their lives the foods and food elements to which they are sensitive. These are called trigger or binge foods: they give people cravings, obsessions, or the inability to stop. Any food can be appropriate in an abstinent food plan, but if a food causes problems for the person, it needs to be removed. Then the food addict is free to use the Twelve Steps to create the life he or she really wants to live.

Often, people have struggled with their obsessions for their whole lives, or since they were very young. Whether they are overweight, normal weight, or underweight, they are all in pain about their relationship with food and eating.

Abusive and compulsive eating have many names and take on many forms: anorexia, bulimia, compulsive overeating, compulsive undereating, abusive restricting, binge-eating disorder, and food addiction. People can move from one form to another. All of these eating disorders have physical, mental, emotional, and spiritual components. I believe that some people have a genetically inherited component; many have parents and siblings or other family members who demonstrate similar problems or related addictions. I've observed that Overeaters Anonymous and its Twelve Step program of recovery provide an effective and compassionate solution for all of these problems. The men and women in OA, who are recovering from their own eating problems, reach out in love to help each other with suggestions, support, and strategies.

This Twelve Step program is spiritual, and it is also a program of action and transformation. It offers the opportunity for relief from obsessive thoughts and abusive behaviors. It offers practical suggestions and people to support the individual's effort to heal and recover.

Physicians, dietitians, therapists, and a variety of other health care professionals have much to offer. But the OA connection gives compulsive eaters the daily support and wisdom they need to follow through consistently on the professional medical recommendations. A sponsor helps his or her sponsee follow the suggestions given; other members listen and offer strategies, support, and a friendly ear. This network of professional and nonprofessional people, and a great deal of compassion and understanding, can empower recovery from eating disorders. I have observed that only those who have learned to effectively use the support of Overeaters Anonymous are able to enjoy long-term recovery and sanity.

Many OA members use an individualized food plan, which is a tool designed to help them know what and when to eat. It is a flexible, usable worksheet that assists with maintaining abstinence from compulsive eating and compulsive food behaviors; it is not a straitjacket or an unreachable goal or standard. An individualized food plan meets the body's nutrient needs, helps to handle medical issues, and meets weight and recovery goals. A food plan should accommodate each person's schedule, food preferences, taste buds, ethnicity, and the reality of life. The food plan should fit the member like a comfortable pair of sneakers. It should be solid, supportive and comfortable enough to help the member travel over the rocky ground of his or her recovery.

It is very important to meet the body's nutrient needs. The body needs the physical support of the nutrients that repair, replace, and maintain its structure and systems. Often, compulsive eaters have used so many restrictive diets in the past that their nutrient needs have not been met for a long time, and the body struggles just to make it through the day—with never enough nutrition.

As part of their plan of eating, some OA members may choose to weigh and measure their food. This can be useful in changing the balance of calories and nutrients in such a way that cravings are diminished and the body has enough to rebuild itself. Achieving the right balance of nutrients is essential for weight loss and maintenance. After years of eating inappropriate amounts of foods, people often have no idea of what the right amount is. It takes time for people to learn to notice when they are hungry, full, or overfull, and then to adjust their food plan appropriately.

Maintaining a healthy weight over the long-term is often harder than losing the weight initially. Once they reach a healthy body size, people must increase their food intake to stop the weight loss, and that can be scary. The joy and delight of losing weight is gone, and the effort of struggling with food, eating, and body weight is gone.

The Twelve Step process teaches the individual a different way of living—a way to create a joyful and useful life without the food obsession. This process must be continued long-term.

Cravings and difficult food situations will continue off and on throughout recovery. This is normal; recovering people need to learn how to handle these issues. They need to plan for times in which they will be confronted with large volumes of food, binge or trigger foods, or difficult food situations. OA provides a range of tools to handle these situations.

Over my years of practice, I have been deeply grateful for the support that members of Overeaters Anonymous have given to my clients. In OA, members have the freedom to create the lives they have dreamed of. They learn how to use the tools and strategies of recovery, and they experience love and support in all of life's challenges.

Nowhere else can people find this kind of training and support, especially not for the simple "fee" of passing it on and helping another member. I wish OA and its members long-term growth and peaceful, joyful recovery.

— *H. Theresa Wright, MS, RD, LDN, 2013*

H. Theresa Wright, a dietitian specializing in addictive and compulsive eating disorders, runs a nutrition center in Pennsylvania. She has helped to carry the OA message in her work with clients and in interviews for an OA Internet radio series. In addition, she reviewed the food plans described in the OA pamphlet *Dignity of Choice*.

APPENDIX B
A Disease of the Mind

Several years ago, as a psychiatrist working in drug abuse and alcoholism programs, I was led, through the experience of a staff member, to examine compulsive overeating as a disease process identical to alcoholism. We started to apply, in a limited fashion, the same principles to the problem of compulsive overeating that we were using in our alcoholism treatment program and found them to be very successful. The more closely I examined the phenomenon, the clearer it became that compulsive overeating is a disease.

In medical school, we doctors are never taught about overeating, certainly not as a disease. So we are prejudiced against it. Overeaters Anonymous is very successful with cases that haven't responded to conventional kinds of treatment. This success is often threatening to the professionals because it's difficult for us to see how someone who hasn't had years of study and experience could be more successful with people we've been trying to treat, unsuccessfully, for so long.

The remarkable thing about OA's success is that the program gets people to function far better than they ever have in their lives. With any other disease, you're lucky to get back to where you were. If you have a heart attack, for example, you're fortunate to get your heart to function as well as it did before the attack.

With the compulsive overeater, not only do you get back to a normal weight, but more importantly, your life is changed, and in a sense, you're ahead of where you were before you became a compulsive overeater. Now you have tools of feeling, touching, caring, loving, sharing, being honest with your family, and looking at life in an understanding way and not fighting it but going along with it. Once you treat the illness, you have the potential to be a more "together" person than you were. Therefore, it's exciting for physicians and others, who have been ignoring the problem or expressing deep pessimism about it, to think of compulsive overeating as a disease and to realize that it can be treated so successfully.

One of the prejudices about compulsive overeating is society's view of a compulsive overeater as someone who is obese. Yet the overeater can be one pound (0.4 kg) overweight or even underweight, as in anorexia nervosa, and still be a compulsive overeater. The illness has nothing to do with weight. That's why it's so silly to go on diets or to weigh all the time.

The problem is with the control of food. Is one preoccupied with controlling food intake to the point that it's interfering with one's life? Just as being an alcoholic is not related to the amount one drinks, being a compulsive overeater is not related to the amount one weighs.

The overeater's problem is not being able to control eating behavior the way other people can, and the need is for a system to control that behavior. Of course, the most effective one is a support system like that of Overeaters Anonymous. What the overeater has to do is turn over the control to a Higher Power. Once it is turned over, the behavior is under control.

A major confusion we in medicine have is the erroneous belief that compulsive overeating is a result of physiologic, psychologic, and environmental problems. We try to treat compulsive overeaters psychiatrically or physically with medicine or structures in their lives, and it doesn't work. The reason it fails is because we are doing it in reverse. What has to be dealt with is the compulsive overeating. When it is, the physiologic and psychiatric problems seem to take care of themselves.

There are some people, about the same percentage as in the general population, who after getting the food back in its proper place, find themselves needing traditional psychiatric care because they do have a problem, which they had pushed down with food. But that is the exception. What is probably true in most cases is that the individual develops the compulsive overeating mechanism for dealing with life at an early age and then starts to push problems down with the food. Once people become compulsive overeaters, every aspect of their lives is affected. Now they get into the psychological, physical, and environmental problems and start changing their lives, their friends, and their social structures. All these changes are really caused by the compulsive overeating. Most compulsive overeaters, through a program like OA's, will lose all these syndromes and not need to have any kind of traditional psychiatric care.

We in the medical community must take responsibility for failing to understand the real problem. Compulsive overeating is a serious disease, and it is devastating this country. It is the basic cause of disorders that medicine views as primary illnesses, such as hypertension and diabetes. But physicians don't look at compulsive overeating, they look at the secondary disease process that comes from compulsive overeating. They ignore the overeating and rigorously work on the symptoms and the secondary diseases.

Obviously, that is not the way to treat it. If a patient has pneumonia, the doctor doesn't treat the fever and then send the patient home after the temperature is normal, saying, "Your fever is down; now watch that pneumonia." But we certainly do this with the overeater. We take care of the symptoms of the secondary disease, and we tell that patient, "Your weight (or blood pressure or blood sugar) is normal; now watch that overeating."

It is the responsibility of the medical community to understand what compulsive overeating really means and to recognize that Overeaters Anonymous has been dealing successfully with the disease. We need to work closely with OA, to have OA as the base or structure, and only then should we offer what we as professionals are able to contribute. The doctor should have the patient go to OA, and then serve as OA's support system for that patient. Overeaters Anonymous should be the treatment, and the professional should be the adjunct, not the other way around. This is very difficult for a physician or mental health professional to accept.

As long as Overeaters Anonymous continues to keep the Principles it has now, it will be our most valuable means of treatment of the disease of compulsive overeating. OA's Principles ensure that no individual has power. In essence, it is a leaderless organization, making the process much stronger than any one member or group.

Overeaters Anonymous is a system of people who are trying to help each other, and as such it is tremendously successful.

— *William Rader, M.D.,*1980

Dr. William Rader is a psychiatrist engaged in clinical work with alcoholism, drug addiction, and compulsive overeating. Winner of the 1977 Appreciation Award of Overeaters Anonymous, he has carried the OA message in his treatment programs.

APPENDIX C
A Disease of the Body

[Note: The statistics quoted below are from 1980, when this appendix was originally published. See the footnote for updated information.]

I was most pleased, several years ago, to be invited as a representative of the American Society of Bariatric Physicians (a medical scientific society devoted to the study of obesity and allied conditions) to attend an annual convention of Overeaters Anonymous. I have since then attended several others. I was also privileged to attend some local group meetings.

The basic concept of Overeaters Anonymous is that compulsive overeating is a disease that affects the person on three levels—physical, spiritual, and emotional. Members of OA feel that, like alcoholics, they are unable to control their compulsion permanently by unaided will power.

Obesity is unquestionably one of the major health problems in the United States today. In fact, it is a problem common to all affluent societies. Estimates as to the number of overweight individuals in the United States range from ten million to more than seventy million, depending on what criteria are used to classify an individual as obese. Furthermore, in recent years there has been a steady increase in the number of overweight individuals. This is due to many factors. Chief among them is our success in creating an abundant food supply while our physical activity continues to diminish.

To indicate the magnitude of this menace, a Gallup Poll in 1973 revealed that 46 percent of Americans polled felt they were overweight, while less than 8 percent thought they were underweight. Out of every ten persons, four or five were doing something to control their weight. Senator George McGovern's committee hearings disclosed that obesity nourishes a ten billion dollar industry, with one hundred million dollars yearly being spent for reducing drugs alone. The US Public Health Service estimates that at least sixty million Americans weigh more than they should. The most disturbing problem is that perhaps less than five percent of dieters are able to maintain weight loss for at least five years.*

As a physician, my main concern with the obese is the medical risks to which their obesity exposes them. Such persons have a

---

* More than one-third of US adults were obese from 2011 to 2012. The estimates for overweight and obesity combined (BMI greater than or equal to 25) were 68.8 percent overall: 73.0 percent among men and 64.7 percent among women. An estimated 18 percent of children ages 6 to 11 and 21 percent of adolescents ages 12 to 19 were obese. (U.S. Department of Health and Human Services, *Health, United States, 2013*, www.cdc.gov/nchs/data/hus/hus13.pdf#064, tables 64, 69)

In 2012, costs associated with obesity accounted for $190 billion annually—121 percent higher than previous estimates. More than 20.6 percent of all national health expenditures is spent on managing obesity and the related plethora of health problems, researchers said. (Amir Khan, *Obesity in America: Healthcare Costs Double Previous Estimates*, Journal of Heath Economics, Vol. 31, Issue 1, Jan 2012, pp. 219-230, www.ibtimes.com/obesity-america-healthcare-costs-double-previous-estimates-435188)

Based on latest available surveys, more than half (53 percent) of the adult population in the Organization for Economic Cooperation and Development (OECD), an international economic organization of thirty-four countries founded to seek answers to common problems and co-ordinate domestic and international policies, report that they are overweight or obese. The prevalence of being overweight and obesity among adults exceeds 50 percent in no less than twenty-one of the thirty-four OECD countries. On average across the OECD countries, 18 percent of the adult population is obese. (*Overweight and obesity*, OECD Factbook 2013: Economic, Environmental and Social Statistics, http://dx.doi.org/10.1787/factbook-2013-100-en)

greater than 40 percent chance of dying in any given year from heart disease, a greater than 30 percent chance of dying from coronary artery disease, a greater than 50 percent death rate from cerebrovascular disease (strokes), as well as an increased death rate from many other diseases. It has also been pointed out recently that the risk of developing diabetes is increased twofold by an increase of 20 percent in body weight. In women, there is also a significant increase in the development of uterine cancer associated with excess body weight. In a recent study of 75,532 fat women, there were sixteen diseases associated with obesity. Furthermore, obesity predisposes to high blood pressure, gallbladder disease, and the formation of gallstones requiring surgery. Even babies born of obese mothers have more than twice the infant mortality of babies whose mothers' weights are normal.

Most individuals who join Overeaters Anonymous are aware of these risks. But, like alcoholics, they are unable to control their compulsion on any lasting basis. They have completely lost faith in life and in themselves. In OA, hands of understanding and strength are extended to them by people who suffer the same compulsion and who are now examples that there is an answer. This probably explains OA's success with the hopeless obese person who has repeatedly failed with the usual methods of weight control. I was particularly impressed with the extreme friendliness and even love between members that was easily observable at meetings.

Many OA members are former participants (and dropouts) of commercial weight control groups. I observed a number of individuals who had been unsuccessful in the commercial organizations, but who had reached and maintained normal weight for a number of years after having joined Overeaters Anonymous. On being asked why they switched organizations, they were quick to inform me that the continual preparation of "free" foods and general preoccupation with food, as sometimes expounded, only kept their food compulsion alive.

When compulsive overeaters realize that they cannot control their eating behavior, they need to accept and depend upon another power—a power acknowledged to be greater than oneself. The interpretation of this power is left to the individual. Many, perhaps most, members of OA adopt the concept of God. But newcomers are merely asked to keep an open mind on this subject and usually they find it is not too difficult to work out a solution to this very personal problem, even if they are atheist or agnostic.

Psychologically, the obese individual is helped to attain a sense of the reality and nearness of a greater power, which replaces one's egocentric nature. Then the person's point of view and outlook will take on a spiritual coloring. Hence, one no longer needs to maintain a defiant individuality but can live in peace and harmony with the environment, sharing and participating freely, especially with other members of the group. This is a great therapeutic weapon that I, a physician who has dealt with obese people for more than twenty-seven years, can appreciate. The obese individual no longer defies, but accepts help, guidance, and control from the outside. As OA members relinquish their negative, aggressive feelings toward themselves and toward life, they find themselves overwhelmed by positive feelings of love, friendliness, tranquility, and a pervading contentment. These latter feelings were evident among the groups I attended.

A word frequently heard in OA groups is surrender. It can best be described as letting go. The individual gives up personal rigidities, relaxes and admits to being beaten by compulsive overeating. The source of this feeling is almost always despair, which is so prevalent in newcomers to the group. It is all part of a crisis experience, with an overload of hopelessness. In the act of surrender, one does not just give up but accepts a power greater than oneself, reducing the ego and admitting the need for outside help.

The "ego reduction" can be very profitable to the personality makeup of this person. It is important to differentiate between submission and surrender. In submission, an individual accepts reality consciously but not unconsciously. There is acceptance that one cannot, at the moment, conquer reality, but lurking in the unconscious is the feeling that "there will come a day when I will be able to handle my problem on my own."

Submission implies no real acceptance of one's inadequacy; on the contrary, it demonstrates conclusively that the struggle is still going on. Submission is, at best, a superficial yielding, with the inner tensions still present. When the individual accepts, on an unconscious level, the reality of not being able to handle compulsive overeating, there is no residual battle. Relaxation ensues with a freedom from strain and conflict. This freedom is the aim of the OA groups, and complete surrender is manifested by the considerable degree of relaxation that is evident in the behavior of those who have achieved it.

Once compulsive overeaters surrender at the unconscious level, their compliance with the disciplines of the program does not lessen with time, leading to the inevitable regaining of weight. They continue to get messages from the unconscious that the need for outside help will remain for a prolonged, if not indefinite, period. Their wholehearted cooperation is then forthcoming, and constructive action takes the place of skin-deep assurances that they will merely comply temporarily until the memory of their suffering and self-pity weakens and the need for compliance lessens.

Surrender, then, is an unconscious event. It is not willed by the individual. It can occur only when one becomes involved with one's unconscious mind in a set of circumstances that signal the undeniable need for an external greater power. The definition of surrender can be understood only when all its unconscious ramifications and true inner meaning are glimpsed. Observed by others, such an individual manifests an inner calm and a "live and let live" attitude.

In analyzing Overeaters Anonymous, I have reached a number of conclusions. There appears to be a deep shift in the individual's emotional tone, the disappearance of one set of feelings and the emergence of a very different set. The member moves from a negative state of mind to a positive one. This may have the earmarks of a spiritual conversion. Be that as it may, it is an effective transformation and essential for long-term success.

By this I do not mean to imply that there are never any slipups.

Indeed, there are. But they are usually due to overconfidence as people are successful in the program and once again become too preoccupied with themselves. As long as they attend group meetings, help is immediately available, inspiring them to return to abstinence and to the Twelve Steps of recovery. They are neither judged nor scolded. There are no weigh-ins. They can share their past experiences, their present problems, and their hopes for the future with those who understand and support them and who speak their own language. Working with a sponsor, the individual converses with a person who has been through similar experiences. Thus the communication between these two is on the same level. When OA members become sponsors themselves, their loneliness is greatly alleviated. They are needed and accepted. This has a very potent, positive influence on weight maintenance.

OA literature suggests that the newcomer visit a doctor to decide upon a plan of eating suited to both physical needs and family habits. I can verify that this was, indeed, the policy with a number of patients whom I have referred to this group. OA is not concerned with the medical aspects of obesity, but with the compulsive nature of overeating.

It is my firm belief that Overeaters Anonymous has made a definite place for itself in helping the obese individual and renders a valuable service to such a person. The empathy and attention individuals receive at meetings during trying times can be of great therapeutic value. Overeaters Anonymous can help individuals restore their faith in themselves and in others and give them hope for recovery. There is no other organization, lay or professional, that has such a profound influence on the compulsive overeater's thinking; and after all, it is our thoughts that precede our emotions, and it is our emotions that make us eat inappropriately and become physically obese. Recovery in OA is on all three levels. It may seem a tall order, but it's one which has the greatest chance for success.

It has been an honor and a most exciting experience for me as a professional to have had the opportunity to get to know the members of Overeaters Anonymous. I will forever be grateful to them for the good work they do in combating a major health problem in the United States.

— *Peter G. Lindner, M.D.*, 1980

Dr. Peter Lindner was past president of the American Society of Bariatric Physicians and chairman of its board of trustees. He received the 1975 Appreciation Award of Overeaters Anonymous in recognition of his work in the field of obesity and compulsive overeating and his efforts to bring the OA program to the attention of the medical community and the general public. Dr. Lindner passed away in 1987.

APPENDIX D
A Disease of the Spirit

The title of this commentary puts in simple words the uniqueness and special place that Overeaters Anonymous has earned and is earning within the whole approach to the problem of compulsive overeating.

It was not easy to determine how to apply a program dealing with alcoholism, in which thousands have learned how to live without drinking, to a commodity—food—without which not one can live. I am sure that this difficulty still exists within the minds of some. For many others, however, it is clear that what compulsive overeaters and alcoholics have in common is a need to nourish the spiritual side of their nature.

All in all, it is the saving grace of the spiritual in the OA program that has made for its success and growth, and I can prophesy that OA will continue to grow, bringing not only sane eating habits but also spiritually and morally oriented lives that will help build society.

Spiritual values are important because they deal with the whole person. Wholeness in this sense is related to "holiness," as well as to "balance." A holy person is one whose body, mind, and spirit share an equality that was (and is) the intention and plan of God for all men. Such a person takes his or her place within the community with ease and grace, motivated by a deep and abiding sense of thanksgiving. Such individuals become creative and constructive, not only with the family circle or community but also in the arts and sciences. Their creative energies are not blocked by shame, guilt, self-pity, and hate or by the facades of arrogance, aggressiveness, and uncaring attitudes.

It is only as the hurt and damaged soul is given emotional and spiritual sustenance that these destructive characteristics slough off, and love begins to flow freely within and from there outward.

Let us look at this spiritual food. To begin with, it falls under the heading of love, the most abused, misused, and yet the most wonderful word in the English language. Without love, every other human virtue or ability is as "sounding brass." Love is a spiritual quality that is not confined to the limits of any religious community. No one has a corner on it. It is free—free to fill the lives of all who allow it to flow freely. And as it flows, it washes and gives life and glorifies its source—God.

This brings me to my first point. Those who are prone to stuff themselves with food that makes their bodies unsightly are refusing the food that satisfies and soothes the unhappy soul within. Have they said, "I don't deserve anything good" for such a long time that they are literally putting their heels on that source of love that alone can bring peace? Or have they become so discouraged or so angry that they deny even the existence of love, let alone God?

All of us can identify with such feelings. Compulsive overeaters and alcoholics, gamblers and drug addicts are not the only inhabitants of life's gray areas. The number of such afflicted people is legion.

There are three stages in the process of getting any kind of food. One: Take your body to the food. Two: Dish it out and eat it. Three: Enjoy it and use the energy it creates. It is the same with spiritual food, food for the soul. Let us look at these three stages.

One: Take your body to the food. Sometimes people become so sick with overeating that the "spiritual food" has to come through one who cares, one who loves. This is God's method. He first loved us. But sometimes he knocks at the door of our lives in the form of a person or a book or magazine article—a thought, a hope.

The knocking is heard but often the door remains shut. Sooner or later, however, it must be opened to allow some kind of help to enter. In most cases, many kinds of "help" have been tried. They all involved money, effort, and disappointment. Finally, the message gets through: Someone cared enough to reach the starving soul. You allow love within your life. You are ready to take your body to spiritual food.

Two: This stage follows closely upon the accomplishment of the first. How surprising to find—and difficult to believe—that all those people at the OA meeting understood your problem and cared about you!

You see, love that is accepted immediately eliminates your aloneness. The only way you can use the word love when you are alone is by loving yourself, and no compulsive overeater does that at first. So it must begin by allowing someone else's love into your life. This very action of including others and being included is food for the soul—the starving waif within the stuffed body.

But the process of love has only begun. Carefully, even suspiciously, you allow a few people closer to your inner self. Through trusting them, even passively, you move closer to love. You may call these individuals foolhardy to love you, but the pain and loneliness drive you to respond. It becomes easier and easier, until you "overlove" and someone lets you down. This happens because immature love tries to possess and control. Then, you may run back into your shell to lick your wounds, and perhaps a few platters in the process. Like a mighty flood, you feel swamped again by that compulsion that once all but destroyed your life. A phone call: an understanding member of OA hears your story and levels with you. Thankfully, there are many who have learned the difference between loving and "over-loving." They are always standing by, ready to help.

What a relief to be on the raft of OA again—that group of people who take you firmly by the hand in love and fellowship.

It is then that you are encouraged to ingest and digest two new kinds of food: First, understanding for your straightjacketed mind.

This comes from OA literature and other sources. Second, you learn that prayer and meditation have a lot to do with satisfying the inner hungry one. Finally, you can listen to the stories you hear at meetings with a deeper insight. You study the Traditions, born out of pain and trial, which have kept a spiritual movement living and growing for nearly seventy years. You learn that others have personal histories more traumatic than yours. You acquire humility. You learn some of the tricks of the trade of wholesome living. And finally you can turn to the healthy sauce of good humor. You can not only laugh at the ridiculous reasoning and situations others go through, but you learn to laugh at yourself also.

Humor is a most important ingredient of love. I think it shakes down the food—now shrinking away—so that you can make room within yourself for others. This is a major step forward because it takes some of the emotional heat (condemnation) off yourself. And what a relief this is!

Fellowship, understanding, and humor—all of them digestible forms of love: food for the soul.

Somewhere along this pathway the spiritual itself becomes real to you. You begin to be aware of mystical qualities that become important and real. Is this the birth of a soul? No, because the soul was not dead. It was only starving, denied, and stifled. Now it moves within, purring with contentment as it begins its lifelong, God-given task of furnishing control, establishing security and, finally, giving purpose. Now you understand what it was that really attracted you to Overeaters Anonymous. Sure, you were impressed by a slim and trim figure. You wanted that, too. But what really caught you was the love, the understanding, the soul qualities that touched you where you really lived, though you may not have been aware of it.

And wonder of wonders, you too become an instrument of love. You doubted that you could meet the needs of others, but soon the people about you began to respond to your love. Now, you have reached the third stage. You are walking on Cloud Nine, only to be tripped up by pride and even a tinge of complacency or arrogance. The power you envied in others is now yours. You must learn to use it without losing your way again.

Sometimes this experience strands us on a stagnant, arid plateau. You may see someone else maturing more rapidly than you. Disillusionment and standstill can result. There is at this crossroads a signpost you cannot miss: "Go deeper with others and with God."

God has provided many other means of fellowship and growth. They too offer soul food. But always remember that your compulsion with food does demand that kind of understanding and experience that members of OA can provide. But now that your body is no longer your master; your mind is beginning to think clearly; and your soul is fed, nurtured, and functioning, you can reconsider those other sources of soul food.

I now leave off my description of this pilgrim's progress that takes us from compulsive overeating to its replacement with food for the soul. It is a journey that leads straight out of self-made prisons and limitations into green pastures where we find many a table spread with wholesome food and a cup that overflows.

— *The Reverend Rollo M. Boas,* 1980

One of OA's earliest supporters, Reverend Rollo Boas was a minister of the Episcopal church and the recipient of OA's 1979 Appreciation Award. He passed away in 1993.

APPENDIX E
To Find Overeaters Anonymous

You can find OA in most cities across the United States and in more than eighty countries worldwide. Most groups maintain telephone directory or online listings under "Overeaters Anonymous."

Many groups also place announcements giving a local telephone contact number in the community listings or in the classified section of newspapers.

If there are no public listings of OA groups in your area or if you need information about OA in other countries, check the website at www.oa.org or write or call the World Service Office, PO Box 44727, Rio Rancho, NM 87174-4727 USA, 1-505-891-2664.

The international headquarters for Overeaters Anonymous, Inc., the World Service Office, maintains up-to-date meeting directories, publishes OA literature, and provides a broad range of other services for groups, intergroups, national and language service boards, and regional offices throughout the world.

APPENDIX F
OA Publications

The World Service Office has over 100 literature items to support you in your program. Go to bookstore.oa.org or contact the World Service Office for more information.

Books

The Twelve Steps and Twelve Traditions of Overeaters Anonymous, Second Edition

The Twelve Step Workbook, Second Edition

For Today and *For Today Workbook*

Voices of Recovery and *Voices of Recovery Workbook*

Abstinence, Second Edition

A New Beginning: Stories of Recovery from Relapse

Seeking the Spiritual Path

Taste of Lifeline

Body Image, Relationships, and Sexuality

Pamphlets

Where Do I Start?

In OA, Recovery Is Possible

Dignity of Choice

A Plan of Eating: A Tool For Living

The Tools of Recovery

Many Symptoms, One Solution

A Lifetime of Abstinence: One Day at a Time

OA Members Come in All Sizes

1. We admitted we were powerless over food—that our lives had become unmanageable.

2. Came to believe that a Power greater than ourselves could restore us to sanity.

3. Made a decision to turn our will and our lives over to the care of God *as we understood Him.*

4. Made a searching and fearless moral inventory of ourselves.

5. Admitted to God, to ourselves and to another human being the exact nature of our wrongs.

6. Were entirely ready to have God remove all these defects of character.

7. Humbly asked Him to remove our shortcomings.

8. Made a list of all persons we had harmed, and became willing to make amends to them all.

9. Made direct amends to such people wherever possible, except when to do so would injure them or others.

10. Continued to take personal inventory and when we were wrong, promptly admitted it.

11. Sought through prayer and meditation to improve our conscious contact with God *as we understood Him,* praying only for knowledge of His will for us and the power to carry that out.

12. Having had a spiritual awakening as the result of these Steps, we tried to carry this message to compulsive overeaters and to practice these principles in all our affairs.

Permission to use the Twelve Steps of Alcoholics Anonymous
for adaptation granted by AA World Services, Inc.

THE TWELVE TRADITIONS OF OVEREATERS ANONYMOUS

1. Our common welfare should come first; personal recovery depends upon OA unity.

2. For our group purpose there is but one ultimate authority—a loving God as He may express Himself in our group conscience. Our leaders are but trusted servants; they do not govern.

3. The only requirement for OA membership is a desire to stop eating compulsively.

4. Each group should be autonomous except in matters affecting other groups or OA as a whole.

5. Each group has but one primary purpose—to carry its message to the compulsive overeater who still suffers.

6. An OA group ought never endorse, finance or lend the OA name to any related facility or outside enterprise, lest problems of money, property and prestige divert us from our primary purpose.

7. Every OA group ought to be fully self-supporting, declining outside contributions.

8. Overeaters Anonymous should remain forever non-professional, but our service centers may employ special workers.

9. OA, as such, ought never be organized; but we may create service boards or committees directly responsible to those they serve.

10. Overeaters Anonymous has no opinion on outside issues; hence, the OA name ought never be drawn into public controversy.

11. Our public relations policy is based on attraction rather than promotion; we need always maintain personal anonymity at the level of press, radio, films, television and other public media of communication.

12. Anonymity is the spiritual foundation of all these Traditions, ever reminding us to place principles before personalities.

Permission to use the Twelve Traditions of Alcoholics Anonymous for adaptation granted by AA World Services, Inc.